Just Here,
Doctor

Just Here, Doctor

Dr Robert Clifford

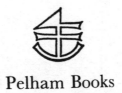

Pelham Books

First published in Great Britain
by White Lion Publishers Ltd, 1977

This edition published in Great Britain by
PELHAM BOOKS LTD
44 Bedford Square
London WC1B 3EF
February 1978
Second impression August 1979

Illustrated by Bill Martin (*Sunday Express*)

ISBN 0 7207 1055 3

Filmset in Great Britain by
Northumberland Press Ltd., Gateshead, Tyne and Wear
and printed by Billing and Son, London, Guildford and Worcester

To my wife, Pam

Prologue

Life is a tragedy, for we are all born eventually to die. We survive our tragedies by laughing at them.

'A friend once told me that when he was under the influence of ether he dreamed he was turning over the pages of a great book, in which he knew he would find, on the last page, the meaning of life.

'The pages of the book were alternately tragic and comic, and he turned page after page, his excitement growing, not only because he was approaching the answer but because he couldn't know, until he arrived, on which side of the book the final page would be. At last it came: the universe opened up to him in a hundred words: and they were uproariously funny.

'He came back to consciousness crying with laughter, remembering everything. He opened his lips to speak. It was then that the great and comic answer plunged back out of his reach.'

Christopher Fry

Contents

I

In Need of Practice

I had begun to hate Winchcombe Hospital. I had nothing against the place itself, but I had been doing residential hospital jobs for three and a half years and was fed up with lack of sleep, lack of time off, and endless, tasteless hospital meals.

I had come to Winchcombe because I had hoped to go into general practice in the area, but here I was with just one month of my year's appointment to go, and no sign of anything on the horizon. Thirty-seven interviews for various practices had seen me on the short list of only six, and each time I had been turned down in favour of a married doctor.

The fact that I had come to Winchcombe after a failed romance did not in any way sweeten my bitter cup.

However, there was still hope. A practice in Tadchester had asked me to come and see them on Sunday. They did not give details, but I knew them all vaguely as I had treated some of their patients. This was hopeful certainly – or would it be another fruitless interview with my precious Sunday off wasted?

There was no direct bus service from Winchcombe to Tadchester on a Sunday, and I had not been able to afford a car on my measly hospital pay, but one of the consultants, John Bowler, kindly lent me his wife's car for the day. I drove off in plenty of time for my three o'clock appointment.

The second half of the drive was along the coast road, and I was watching some yachts out at sea as I drove along.

My reverie was interrupted by a screeching of brakes and the shattering of glass. Oh God! I slammed on my brakes and jumped out of the car to find an irate woman of about thirty-five examining the side of her car. I had drifted into her as she was about to pass me, and taken the side almost completely off.

She was furious.

'You damned fool,' she shouted. 'Were you asleep? Don't you ever look out of your rear mirror?'

We exchanged names and addresses. She was a Mrs Jean Hart of Tadchester. Fortunately both cars were still roadworthy, and I drove on, shaken, wondering how I was going to tell John Bowler about the crumpled wing and battered sidelight of his car. It just didn't look like being my day.

I reached Tadchester at about 2.30, parked outside the surgery of Drs Maxwell, Johnson and Hart, and rang the bell. There was no reply, so I sat in the car waiting for somebody to open up.

By three o'clock nobody had appeared. I got out and walked round the surgery to the back where there were living quarters, and saw a caretaker's bell which I pressed. Again there was no reply, so I went back to the car and fished out the letter confirming their phone call. The address right enough, was 'Drs Maxwell, Johnson and Hart, The Surgery, Tadchester'. Then my heart sank. The letter said that the appointment would be at Dr Johnson's house, Hillsborough House, The Hill, Tadchester.

I leapt into the car, asked directions from a passer-by, and eventually – at 3.45 – arrived at a huge house at the top of the hill, the other side of the River Tad from where I had been waiting at the surgery.

I ran to the door, out of breath. I was met by a very tall, thin, gruff man, whose greeting was 'You are late. I am Dr Johnson. Come in. We have been waiting for you.'

I was taken in and introduced to the other two doctors, both of whom looked stern and impatient. The shorter one I gathered was Dr Maxwell, and the red-haired one was Dr Hart.

Dr Maxwell, who seemed a kindly man, said, 'We have

interviewed twelve people in the last two days: you are the only one who has kept us waiting.'

My heart dropped. Twelve. And I bet they were all married. What chance did I stand?

They asked a few perfunctory questions. I thought they were just going through a few polite motions before they turfed me out. They did seem to know quite a bit about me, and we discussed some of their cases I had coped with at Winchcombe Hospital. They obviously knew John Bowler, my physician, very well.

The tension that had been in the room earlier lessened. We were chatting amicably about cases when Dr Maxwell, with a smile on his face, said, 'Now is the hardest part of the interview. Come and meet the partners' wives. There are only two; I, like yourself, have remained independent.'

There was one of those awkward pauses when all four of us

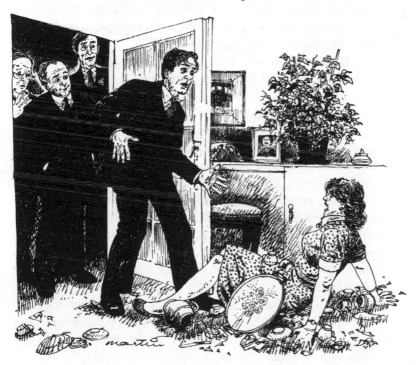

were standing back to let the others go through the door first. Eventually, I stepped forward and pushed the door open. It hit something and there was the most resounding crash. On the floor behind the door was a lady and the wreckage of a tray of tea. I helped her up, apologising profusely, and vaguely aware that I recognised her.

'My God,' she said, 'it's the maniac driver! What the hell are you doing here?'

This was all I needed.

The name 'Hart' should have rung a bell. Of all the people I could have crashed into in my reverie I had to choose the wife of one of the men who were interviewing me. I daren't look at the cups and saucers on the floor – they were bound to be part of a best bone china set that had been in the family for two hundred years.

My slight hope of being selected flew out of the window.

Another lady, obviously Mrs Johnson, came out to help clear up and organise a further tea.

The three partners and I sat waiting for the two ladies in a gloomy silence. Dr Maxwell tried to make light conversation, but nobody took him up.

Eventually the ladies joined us and tea was conducted in a chilly silence. Mrs Johnson, the wife of the tall, thin man, was obviously very refined. She questioned me about my school and background, neither of which appeared to impress her over-much. I had been to grammar school, not a public school. I did not ride, had no money, and was badly dressed.

Somehow we got through tea. Dr Maxwell, whom I liked best, saw me to the door and said, 'We have one or two more candidates to see, but we'll be in touch.'

I had heard all this before. Sadly I got into the battered car and drove back to Winchcombe.

John Bowler laughed when I told him my experiences.

'Don't you worry, Bob,' he said, 'I think the job is yours. And don't worry about the car: it's covered by insurance.' I just couldn't believe him.

Two days later I was rung by Dr Johnson saying that I had been selected and that they wanted me to start next week as an assistant for six months with a view to partnership. At last I had found a practice.

I told him I would be delighted to join them but had one further month to do of my hospital appointment to complete it, then I would be able to start on the first of the next month.

Dr Johnson replied very sternly, 'You either come next week or not at all,' and slammed the phone down.

I was furious. Going into partnership was like getting married. I would probably spend the rest of my life with these people. How could he speak to me like this? And what would the hospital do? They wouldn't release me. I had to serve my time out.

I took all my troubles to John Bowler.

'Bob,' he said, 'take my advice. These are fine doctors. They are at their wits' end in the middle of a 'flu epidemic. They have had all sorts of partner trouble which I won't go into, but I wouldn't be advising you to go unless I thought they were a good practice.

'They are worn out, they are weary – and they need you. Leave it to me to sort things out with the hospital. My advice is go – if you have problems you can always come over and weep on my shoulder.'

So I was to go into practice at last. I didn't really believe it, and the circumstances could have been better, but I trusted John Bowler. I sorted out my duties as best I could with my fellow housemen, packed what few belongings I had, and made arrangements to buy my own car.

I knew very little about Tadchester. My only visit had been that disastrous interview. I wondered what Tadchester was going to think of me.

2

A Town like Tadchester

Tadchester is a small town (population 6,500) on the estuary of the River Tad in one of the most beautiful parts of the Somerset coast. It is a Jack-of-all-trades market town, with some fishing, some light industry and a lot of farming.

Six miles north is Thudrock Colliery, known locally as Siberia, where the town's unfortunates are sent by the Labour Exchange if they can't find any other job. As well as the Labour Exchange conscripts, Thudrock employs a good number of men from the town who are miners by choice and heritage.

Tadchester is also a seasonal holiday town and is invaded by holidaymakers from all over the country, particularly from the north. It is 200 miles from London, far enough for people to feel they have really got away. Some of the locals obviously hibernate during the winter, as the summer months bring forth a crop of Tadchester characters who disappear completely once the weather starts to deteriorate.

The town is split in two by the River Tad, and further split by the large hill which dominates one side of the river. The other side is flat pastureland stretching off to marshes and the sea coast. You are not just a Tadchester resident, you are either 'Up the Hill' or 'Down the Hill'.

There is no strict social division between Up the Hill and Down the Hill, but the majority of the down-the-hillers are the

Haves, and the majority of the up-the-hillers are the Have-nots.

The bridge joining the opposite sides of the river is the famous old Tadchester Bridge. People come from miles to walk the bridge and enjoy the view from it, which is one of the best in the area. Quite often the lifeboat from the nearby seaside village of Sanford-on-Sea has actually to come inland to rescue inquisitive children who have toppled over the parapet into the depths of the Tad. In fact, holidaymakers are the only people one ever sees on the bridge – any inhabitant of Tadchester who is seen to cross from one side to the other is immediately branded as a traitor by his neighbours. Old Mr Clegg, who had lived Up the Hill all his life, was once seen by watchful fishermen to sneak across to the Down the Hill side late at night for some undoubtedly furtive reason. His papers and mail weren't delivered for a week.

Luckily, doctors were given carte blanche as far as the bridge was concerned, and I was at liberty to spend the whole day crossing from one side to the other without fear of having my essential services cut off.

By the time I actually did arrive in the practice the 'flu epidemic was past its peak and life had settled to its normal hectic pace.

I liked the look of my three partners: Dr Steve Maxwell, Dr Henry Johnson, and Dr Jack Hart. They were all different. The senior partner, Steve Maxwell, was a saint of a man, a bachelor, and I have never met his equal. His whole life was medicine. There was never too little time for him to go and see anyone or to attend to someone. Whereas we had a rota for weekends off, he worked every Sunday. He was a good listener, thought my jokes were uproarious, could tell some very good yarns of his own (all of which I took with a pinch of salt), and was never far away when help and counselling were needed.

The only time I ever knew Steve other than his usual cheerful self was when a professional lady cellist in her late sixties returned to Tadchester. I gathered she had given him trouble before she had left the area. She pursued Steve from dawn till dusk. If she was going out, she would ring and tell him so; when she got there, she would ring to say that she had arrived, for no particular reason, presumably just to keep in touch. Poor Steve appeared to wilt before us; I had never seen him in this sombre mood before. We were at a loss about how to deal with it.

We had made it a ritual for all four of us to meet every morning for coffee. These were good-humoured gatherings and served a useful purpose, allowing us to blow off steam and share our worries and discuss medical problems. It had become my lot to tell some new outrageous story each day.

Coffee breaks were not the same with Steve in this sort of mood, which seemed to be going on and on. One morning as he stared gloomily into his coffee, I dared to ask, 'How's the cello going, Steve?' He grunted, not looking up.

'You know the real problem,' I said. 'She wants you to pluck her G string.'

Steve collapsed in a fit of laughter that I thought might have developed into hysterics, but it restored his balance, and he was with us once more.

My second partner, Henry Johnson, was the most unflappable man I have ever met; he was also one of the tallest and thinnest. He did the surgery at the local cottage hospital and combined his practice with surgical out-patients' sessions, surgical lists and, in the summer, seemed to live almost day and night at the hospital, dealing with road traffic accidents and the many mishaps that befell the visitors.

Henry had one weakness – he was prone to attacks of crippling lumbago. In his stubborn, dogmatic way, he refused to let it interfere with his work. One afternoon he hobbled painfully in to conduct his ante-natal clinic in spite of our protests that he should be at home in bed. 'Go on,' he growled, 'I can manage.'

The first patient he interviewed comfortably from his desk, telling her to slip behind the screen and prepare for examination. As he got up from his chair to conduct his examination, he twisted, slipped, and fell on the floor. He couldn't move.

'Quick. Help me!' he shouted.

The young lady patient dashed from behind the screen and the

18

two of them struggled, wrestling together to get him up off the floor. It seemed to go on for ages. Eventually they managed to get him sitting on the edge of the examination couch.

'Thank you,' said Henry, the sweat streaming down his face.

At that moment he turned to look properly at his anxious helper, to find that she was absolutely stark naked. They looked at each other and both burst out laughing.

Jack Hart was my third partner. He was a soft-spoken Scot, had a great sense of humour, and did most of the anaesthetics at the hospital. The only time he gave me any cause for concern was on one rare occasion when he was sick and I was looking after him. He had a very painful renal colic; that is, he had a small stone in his kidney. His pain was so great that I gave him an injection of pethidine.

His wife was out at the time but there was no cause for alarm. A kidney stone is a mechanical condition which usually rights itself, and he could come to no harm. My complacency was shattered by a hysterical phone call half an hour later from his wife, Jean, who had just got back from a meeting.

'Where is Jack?' she asked. 'He isn't in the house and his dressing gown is still here.'

Oh God, I thought – he has reacted to his injection and flipped.

I rushed round to his house, to find the wanderer returned and Jean sobbing in the chair; I couldn't tell whether they were sobs of grief, relief or joy. Eventually she recovered sufficiently to explain.

Having put down the phone after speaking to me, she had looked out of the window to see Jack walking up the drive in the rain, in his gumboots and pyjamas, flashing a torch. She feared then that he had really gone. But what had happened was that Jack's next-door neighbour had come knocking frantically at the door. His child had swallowed a penny and was choking: could Jack come straight away? Jack had jumped out of bed straight into his wellies, and rushed round, grabbing his torch en route, to give first aid in his pyjamas.

Jean had recovered by now so we celebrated Jack's return from cuckoo-land with a tot of whisky each. Jack, smiling and quite unperturbed, said, 'I think I have passed my stone. Do you think we have found a new cure?'

I acted as house surgeon when Henry Johnson had his gall bladder out. He didn't really trust any other surgeon except himself and I think he would really have liked to have done it himself with a spinal anaesthetic and a mirror. He made an uninterrupted recovery from his operation until he was convalescing in Spain. While he was out swimming, his stitches burst, and he had to be rescued by the local life guards.

'Lot of rubbish,' said Henry. 'I wouldn't have sunk – I had my finger over the hole.'

I came to the practice armed to the teeth with knowledge of the latest procedures – I was determined to show my colleagues how good and up to date I was. It took only a few weeks in practice to disillusion me completely. All my newly learnt techniques and modern methods were of no avail; my patients had a medical folklore of their own and it was I who had to do the relearning and readjust my way of thinking.

One of the first cases was a man with severe diarrhoea. To the amazement of my partners I was bustling around, sending samples off to laboratories, doing blood tests, determined to make a show of this, my first real test. They watched with interest.

All my tests came back negative. My patient, after a few really stormy and dehydrating days, recovered and went back to work. It was only some months later, when I got to know his wife, that I learnt the true cause of the diarrhoea.

The couple had only been married a few weeks when I was first called to the husband. They were still in a state of bliss, getting to know each other, still somewhat shy, and both wary of saying or doing anything indelicate.

The wife knew the husband was severely constipated, but this was far too delicate a condition to discuss together. Trying to do her best for her man, she fed him with a chocolate laxative in the back row of the cinema. She became so engrossed in the film that she gave him three whole bars and even had a couple of pieces herself. He, poor lad, thought he was enjoying the genuine plain dark bitter.

The wife begged me to keep her secret, and this was one of many confidences I had to tuck away.

After a few months in practice I wondered how my partners had managed to cope before I came. There was no doubt that the patients wanted my services: their appreciation was marked by the flow of goods and produce – eggs, chickens, clothes, joints of meat, and drink – that were showered on the surgery doorstep for me.

It was only later that I realised that any new face appearing was always a sign for all the old lags to come and pour out their endless symptoms which my senior partners had got tired of listening to. The showers of gifts were not because they thought I was such a good doctor but because I looked so hard-up and undernourished, which was a fairly accurate diagnosis.

I had come from being a penniless student to being a penniless doctor with a car to buy, accommodation to find, as well as having to put some money into a share of the practice equipment. This did not leave any cash for the replacement of my frayed shirts, tattered trousers and jackets, very much worn down at the elbows.

I reminded my grandfather that ten years previously he had said that, if I ever became a doctor, he would lend me some money to buy a car. Otherwise I would have been doing my visits on a bicycle. Grandfather had made this promise in the perfect confidence that I would never qualify at anything, and required a lot of cajoling before he actually came up with the goods.

My impoverishment was highlighted when, for a time, we had an assistant. Although he was just as poor as I was, he had inherited a very smart black overcoat from his father. On his first visit, with a flashy case and his smart coat, he was answered at the door with 'Not today, thank you – we have got somebody ill in here.'

Nobody gave him anything. He was envious of the piles of

goodies that I seemed to accumulate all the time. At last, one day, he came in triumphant, with a single egg clasped in his right hand like the torch of the Olympic runner.

'You see, I *am* wanted,' he cried.

'Who gave you that?' I asked, jealous of his success.

'Nobody,' answered our assistant. 'There was a bowl of eggs on the table at my last visit and I pinched one.'

Medical school had not prepared me for most of the conditions I had to deal with, and I found it very difficult to communicate with my patients. A young Irish girl came in, obviously seven or eight months gone, complaining of a swollen stomach.

'What do you think it is, doctor?'

'Is there any chance that you could be pregnant?' I asked.

'I was,' said the girl, blushing, 'but I killed the baby.'

She pulled up her dress to show a piece of Elastoplast stuck across her navel.

'I stopped it breathing.'

She did not appear again, but six months later I had a piece of christening cake with an Eire stamp on the packet. The enclosed card said 'With love from Kathleen'. Obviously her faith in Elastoplast had been dispelled.

My Irish girl's lack of knowledge was surpassed only by another lady who arrived, excited, at my ante-natal clinic, having been threatening to come for several weeks, saying she was pregnant. Before examining her I was trying to work out when she was likely to be due.

'When was your last period?' I asked.

'Oh, I've got one now, doctor,' she said. 'You won't be able to examine me until it has stopped ...'

I was once nearly electrocuted by a delightful old vicar who lived with his sister at the far end of the practice. He was lying in bed at home when I saw him for the first time. When I touched his wrist to take his pulse, I had what felt very much like an electric shock. And every time the metal end of my stethoscope got within an inch of his chest, sparks began to fly across the intervening space.

'Whatever else is wrong with you,' I said, 'you are full of electricity. I will have to earth you before I can examine you.'

There had been no mention of this situation during my medical training. I got a piece of wire from his workshop, tied it round his ankle, took the other end out of the window and stuck it in the ground round a six-inch nail. I completed my examination without electrical interference and then took the earth wire off. As soon as I had removed the wire, I got a shock again whenever I touched him. Not only was he the most electric man I had ever come across, but he seemed to be an expert at recharging his own batteries.

I had to call in the Electricity Board for a second opinion. A brisk man in a deerstalker cap assessed the situation and said, 'The explanation is quite simple. He is lying on an electric blanket that has been wired round the wrong way. Even when it has been turned off it acts as a condenser.'

I took the precaution from then on of wearing rubber-soled shoes whenever I went visiting.

I had become very friendly with Eric Martin, the proprietor of the Tadchester Electrical Services. He had a shop in Bridge Street, just 200 yards from the river. We used to go about a lot together and often, on a Wednesday when we both had the afternoon off, would go in search of a rugby match. A few days after my electrical excitement with the vicar, he produced an electronic screwdriver.

'Just the thing for your medical case,' he said. 'If you find any more electric patients, touch them with this and the handle should light up.'

I had only a few weeks to wait to use it. One crusty, retired, old Army officer, Colonel Langston – a private patient – had been in bed for a week with bronchitis. He spent the whole week roasting, with his electric blanket turned full on. He was too comfortable. He had a TV set at the foot of the bed, he smoked incessantly (spilled ash all over the sheets), and I thought we would never get him up.

I had an odd tingle when I examined him, and thought that

23

this was the time to try out my new instrument. First I examined his chest with my stethoscope. It was absolutely clear, but I did allow myself a 'tut-tut'.

'What is it?' he asked. 'I thought I was improving.'

I reached into my bag, pulled out my screwdriver and put the point on his chest. To my delight, the fluorescent tube in the handle glowed. I repeated this about six times, with the Colonel's eyes almost popping out of his head.

'You are getting too much electricity,' I said. 'You will have to get up.'

He was out of bed and beginning to get dressed before I had finished packing my medical case.

I had an odd tingle on one other occasion, when called to visit the local beauty queen – Gwendoline Jacobs – who was complaining of tonsillitis.

She met me at the door in the smallest bikini I have seen, and lay on a black satin-covered couch for me to conduct my examination. I got the same shock when I touched her, but no sparks when I pulled out my stethoscope.

'What a pity,' said my beaming patient, 'that your stethoscope doesn't have shorter tubes.'

'Roll over,' I said quickly, and plunged a syringe full of penicillin into a bronze buttock. I had the feeling that if I were not careful my rubber-soled shoes were going to let me down.

Gwendoline rubbed her buttock ruefully. 'I would like a good over-haul, doctor,' she said, 'a really full check-up.'

'I am afraid we don't have time to do that on the National Health Service,' I replied. 'The only time we do full examinations of fit people is for insurance companies.'

I grabbed my case and bolted.

Gwendoline came off the couch at speed to detain me, but her penicillin-filled bottom pulled her up with a jolt.

I made the front door safely. Gwendoline was left standing, with one hand on the couch taking the weight off her puncture.

'Can you recommend a good insurance company?' she shouted.

24

I closed the front door behind me.

*   *   *

I was called to see Mrs Southern, the wife of a local solicitor. Mr Southern was a precise, meticulous man who liked everything in order and wanted everything explained in detail. The fact that he did not understand medicine meant nothing to him: he was quite prepared for me to spend an hour explaining to him in detail exactly what might be wrong with him or his wife, and all the possible permutations of what it could be, what it might be, and what it could lead to. 'I have a right to know, doctor,' he would say.

I was puzzled by Mrs Southern, who was obviously dominated by her husband. She had giddy attacks and occasionally would collapse. She needed quite some rousing after one of her collapses, which were attended by spells of sleepiness that I could find no explanation for. I did routine blood tests and routine urine tests. There was no sign of her being diabetic. I thought she was rather thin and wondered whether she ate enough, but just could not pin down what might be wrong with her.

Her illness was episodic. She might be perfectly well all day, then I would be called by her husband in the evening to another of her attacks.

He was getting more and more impatient with my failure to diagnose, and made the observation that during her attacks, when she was slurry and confused, there was often a strong formalin-like smell about her.

I looked round their tidy house, precise and clean, like Mr Southern's shirt and tie, the row of Bibles on the shelf (they were staunch churchgoers) and wondered if she could possibly be drinking too much.

I ventured to question Mr Southern about this possibility and was met with an indignant blast of rage – how dare I suggest such a thing! Neither he nor his wife ever touched a drop: there was, in fact, no drink in the house.

25

I was called twice more to see Mrs Southern, in what I now called a 'slurry attack' where she could hardly stand up and was sleepy and muddled.

'Well,' I said, 'when she has her next attack, I want you to collect a specimen of her urine during her attack or as close to it as possible, and bring it round to the surgery.'

The police were very good at estimating the amount of alcohol in people's urine: why shouldn't I be?

A few days later Mr Southern came round with a specimen.

'She has had one of her attacks again, doctor. I am extremely worried, and I do hope you find something from whatever tests you are doing on her water.'

I sent her specimen to the Winchcombe Path. Lab., asking for a urine alcohol estimation as soon as possible.

The pathology technician rang me back a few hours later. My suspicion was right. Her urine was full of alcohol. She was a secret drinker. As the cheery technician said on the telephone, 'I shouldn't stand with a lighted match too close to anyone passing this stuff, doctor – they are likely to blow up.'

I had to go to the Southerns, take Mr Southern out on his own and gently explain to him that there was no doubt that his wife was drinking a lot of alcohol. He was absolutely flabbergasted and just couldn't believe it. He was also deeply hurt and upset, and I comforted him as best I could.

'I know she can't be drinking, doctor,' he said. 'There just isn't any drink anywhere.'

'Let me know one day when she is out,' I said, 'and we'll search the house together.'

Southern consented. 'This sounds awful – going behind my wife's back – but her health's at risk. She is getting steadily worse.'

A few days later his wife was out and together we ransacked the house. Mr Southern found the treasure trove: at the back of the airing cupboard there were twenty-seven empty cooking-sherry bottles.

Mrs Southern was the first of many lonely housewives I found who comforted themselves with sherry that only too often became consumed in increasing quantities.

In those days you could get cooking sherry for about five shillings a bottle, and you didn't have to go to a wine shop or pub to buy it. Cooking sherry could always be put on the grocer's bill, and this was the hidden source from which it came.

We had to confront Mrs Southern with her terrible secret, and Mr Southern had to look into himself to see that perhaps he had become far too concerned with his own interests and just accepted his wife as an uncomplaining housekeeper.

Happily, in their case, the matter resolved itself. Mrs Southern was able to kick the habit, and from then on she and her husband knew each other better and enjoyed each other more.

Unfortunately this was not always the case. Sometimes the first I knew about a secret sherry drinker was when a patient (usually a lady patient) appeared with a liver damage that was almost beyond repair.

3

All Things to All Men

Our practice was run from a central surgery near the centre of the town. There was another branch surgery to cope with the few miners who lived in the terraced cottages .near Thudrock Colliery. We all, in turn, paid it one visit each week.

The branch surgery was very primitive: a disused garage with a row of coloured medicine bottles with a simple dispensing formula upon each bottle: 'One part of medicine to ten parts of water'. I never knew what was in the bottles but most of the patients knew whether they wanted the green or the red or the yellow medicine. They all seemed.fit and healthy, so who was I to argue?

As the only practice in Tadchester we not only coped with all the ills of the local populace, but also ran the cottage hospital. There we became surgeons, surgical assistants or anaesthetists, and sometimes perming any two from three.

I had worked for a couple of years in a large London hospital where there was a constant battle. The general practitioners tried to get rid of their patients by sending them into hospital. The hospital doctors tried to get rid of their patients by sending them back to their general practitioners. At Tadchester I found myself totally committed. After I had sent a patient into hospital, I had to look after him when he got there. If I did kick anybody out of the hospital, I had to look after him when he got home.

I still found my patients difficult to treat. One day I was called to see Granny Branch who lived in a tenement Up the Hill. I made an instantaneous and confident diagnosis, even though I was becoming more wary of doing this.

Granny Branch was lying in a stinking bed. She was covered in sores on her lower abdomen, was desperately thirsty, and a bit confused – clearly a case of diabetes. I had been taught as a medical student never to initiate treatment until I had confirmed the diagnosis, so I asked her daughter to bring a specimen of Granny's urine down to the surgery as soon as she could.

To my surprise the specimen was clear and inoffensive. To my greater surprise it didn't contain any sugar, and sugar was needed to confirm the diagnosis.

I went to bed troubled, calling round early the next day to find Granny Branch deeply unconscious; the family had not bothered to tell me because they knew I was coming. I rushed her into hospital and found that she was in severe diabetic coma – my original diagnosis. I received a tongue lashing from the house surgeon who asked why I hadn't tested her urine, which was loaded with sugar.

This didn't make sense. I called in on Martha, her daughter, and asked her had it been difficult getting a specimen from Granny.

'Well, doctor,' said Martha, hesitantly, 'you did say you must have a specimen of water or Gran might become very ill. I couldn't wake her up properly to get one, so I brought you some of mine.'

This was awful. Not only had I failed my patient, but now I'd got a bad name at the hospital. Was I going to be wrong with every diagnosis I made? Could even Mrs Jenkins be fooling me in some obscure way?

Mrs Jenkins was a patient who lived in an isolated cottage with a large vegetable garden in the flat pastureland of Down the Hill. I was called to see her because she was yellow. There were two possible diagnoses – she could only have either an infection of her liver, or gall bladder trouble. She seemed surprisingly well and untroubled by her colour, and the blood tests I had taken should have given a clear diagnosis of either gall bladder or liver trouble.

She was surprisingly active, carrying on with her housework and looking like a vigorous Chinese coolie. Doubts were beginning to cross my mind, so I rang the Path. Lab. All the blood tests were clear. Her blood was perfectly normal with no evidence of jaundice. Surely I couldn't have sent the wrong blood by mistake? In this case, I was certain her daughter hadn't slipped me hers because I had actually stuck the needle in myself.

I went back to the yellow Mrs Jenkins.

'How are you?' I asked.

'Fine, doctor,' she said.

'What is your appetite like?'

'Fine, doctor,' she said.

'Is there any food that you usually like that you don't like now?' (This was a leading question as people with gall bladder and liver upsets usually develop an aversion to fatty foods.)

'No, doctor.'

'Well, what did you have for lunch today?'

'I had a few carrots,' said Mrs Jenkins.

This was harmless enough and certainly healthy enough, even if a little strange.

'And what are you going to have for dinner tonight?'

'I think I might have a few more carrots.'

Slowly something began to dawn.

'Did you have carrots yesterday Mrs Jenkins?' I asked.

'Oh, yes, doctor.'

'And I expect you will have a few tomorrow?'

'Yes,' said the smiling patient.

I looked out on the large garden. If I had only taken notice of the whole of the patient's environment. The garden was planted with what seemed endless rows of carrots. Mrs Jenkins had carrotaemia – a pigment developed from eating too many carrots.

'How many carrots do you eat a day, Mrs Jenkins?' I enquired.

'Oh, usually about seven pound, doctor.'

'And what happens when they run out in the garden?' I asked.

'I keep a few in stock,' said Mrs Jenkins, opening a tallboy that was crammed from top to bottom with tins of carrots.

During the war, she told me, everybody had been encouraged to eat carrots and she had got a taste for them, tinned carrots being one of the few things in plentiful supply. Yes, she had noticed that she was getting a bit yellow but it had not bothered her; she thought it must be sunburn.

Another failure!

'I see awfully well in the dark,' she said as I trudged wearily to my car.

After Mrs Jenkins I resigned myself to the fact that if I considered every case to be abnormal, occasionally something straightforward would come up to confuse me. I didn't have to wait long.

To finish off a recovering tonsillitis I gave the patient some Mendells paint to paint his throat with. This was a sticky substance which cut down the soreness of swallowing. It is little used nowadays and has been replaced by sophisticated lozenges.

On my enquiring about the throat a week later, the patient said, 'Fine, but I find my shirt keeps sticking to my neck.'

He had painted the *outside* of his neck, and had so gummed up his clothing that he was thinking of sending me his laundry bill.

A child who had an allergic runny nose I treated with antihistamine nasal drops. There was a good response, so I said to the parents, 'I think we should now try and treat the condition with antihistamine tablets.' Two days later I was met by a furious mother and father who said, 'We want to see Dr Maxwell and have some proper treatment. Since we have been putting these tablets up Jenny's nose she can't breathe!'

My final call one Saturday afternoon was to a hunt accident. A very superior young lady in an immaculate white Land Rover and with an accent that matched her white teeth and breeches said, 'Come with me quickly, doctor! One of the hunt's come off his 'orse!'

Grabbing my bag, I jumped into the Land Rover. We bumped

across rutty fields into some woods to where two horses were tethered.

'We ride from here, doctor,' she said.

I hate horses. I once rode a camel quite successfully, but horses terrify me. And horses are like dogs – if they know you are terrified, they do their best to make the condition worse.

That horse was at least thirty feet high – I certainly seemed miles off the ground. I clung round his neck, forgetting my dignity, gripping as best I could with my knees. We covered the first stubble field successfully, but as my mount soared over the first hedge I became detached and crashed down into the ditch.

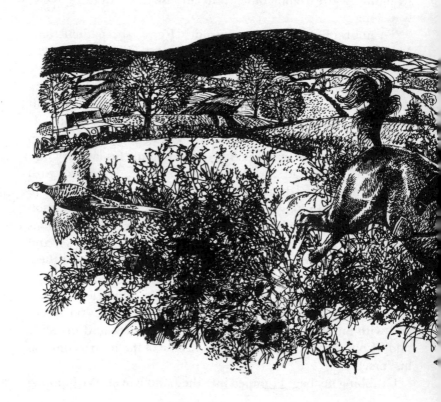

I had an awful pain in my back. My legs were not broken – I could move them – but apart from them I felt that every other bone in my body must have gone at least twice. I was covered in mud. At least it felt like mud, but smelt very much like an old farmyard.

By now the whole of the hunt had assembled around me. The man I had been called to see had recovered and helped to lift me back into the Land Rover. They drove me back to the surgery and with the aid of the grinning Jack Hart they laid me gently on the examination couch. The expression of the buck-toothed young lady who had originally picked me up had not changed

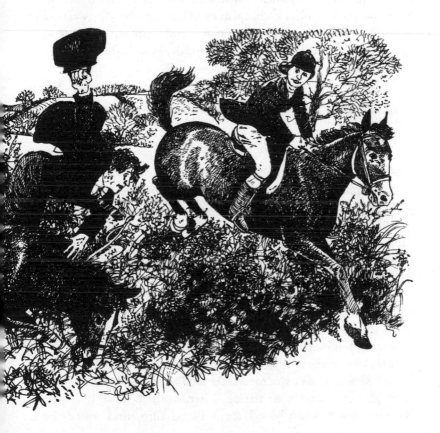

during the whole of our afternoon's companionship. As she left to go, she turned at the door and said, 'Thank you for coming so promptly, doctor. I don't think we appreciate our doctors enough.'

I was three days off with my back. My surgical partner, Henry, just couldn't understand it. If he had hurt his back he would have slapped a quick plaster jacket on himself and carried on. I wasn't made of such stern stuff.

My prompt attendance at the hunt became my introduction to the Upper Crust. I had made an impression on them; they had certainly made an impression on me, or at least my back. My guide with the teeth and tight-fitting breeches turned out to be Marjorie de Wyrebock, daughter of Commander de Wyrebock, R.N. Retd, a local gentleman farmer and a prominent patron of many local events. I was not at ease dealing with these sort of people.

As Mrs de Wyrebock informed me on one of my visits, when she was younger, the doctor was always admitted through the tradesmen's entrance. How democratic everyone had become nowadays.

Commander de Wyrebock was a fine, tall, rather deaf old man. Eight years previously he had been operated on for abdominal pain and at the operation was found to have a cancer of the pancreas gland. It was considered inoperable, his abdomen closed, since when he had had no more trouble and lived, apart from his deafness, a perfectly full, normal life. Just one more example to show that the people in this practice were quite different from those anywhere else.

I was once summoned to see Mrs de Wyrebock when she had a severe headache and fever. Her eyes were a bit puffy. She also claimed that her nose was a bit blocked. I had a good look at her and thought, again unguardedly, this was going to be simple: obviously sinusitis. Because of my uneasiness with the Upper Crust, I over-doctored. As well as giving her antibiotics, antihistamines and nose drops, I arranged to have her sinuses X-rayed, took some blood for a blood film, and asked for a specimen of urine to be sent to the surgery. I speculated on what the specimen would arrive in – probably a jewelled snuff box, at the very least a sterilised whisky decanter. It was sometimes difficult to believe that these people had to follow the calls of nature like us ordinary mortals.

I was asked – commanded – to see two other people on the farm while I was there – Janice, the wife of Kevin Bird, the farm manager, and one of the herdsmen, Bill Foulkes. Janice and Kevin were great friends of mine and I often went round there for meals. They were determined to marry me off and produced a series of possible mates, dragging me off to parties and dances with the usual, 'We think we have found someone you will really like to make up the party.'

I found that Janice had very much the same symptoms as Mrs de Wyrebock. She looked awful, trying to put a brave face on things, but had puffy eyes and a terrible headache and was running a temperature.

To my great surprise I found Bill Foulkes was complaining of exactly the same things as my two previous patients. I was always wary of Bill. He was such an old lead-swinger that he had everything that was going. However, like the other two, he had a temperature and swelling round the eyes, so I could not ignore the symptoms. There had been a high pollen count for the last two days and it did not seem unreasonable that three people associated with the farm should have high fever and sinusitis.

I now regretted having been so over-meticulous with Mrs de Wyrebock. I always considered myself a sort of working-class doctor with the same treatments for everybody, so Janice and Bill Foulkes got the same treatment as their employer's wife. They had antibiotics, antihistamines, nose drops, X-rays arranged, and blood samples taken. All three were National Health Service patients so I had to see everything was even.

The de Wyrebocks, although obviously wealthy, looked for everything that was given for nothing. Being a National Health patient was democratic, like letting your doctor in through the

35

front door. They still of course expected private treatment as National Health Service patients. You felt that they thought they were doing you a favour by asking you to call.

This was a battle I was going to have to fight in future, but I resolved to have Mrs De Wyrebock queueing in the surgery one day for the repeat prescription for sleeping pills she always demanded should be sent round.

I called back to see my patients three days later, rather smugly looking forward to the welcome I would receive for having worked magic cures. Sinusitis is a miserable condition and I had found if you hit it hard at the beginning with nose drops, anti-histamines and antibiotics, the cure was often dramatic.

My first call was, of course, at the de Wyrebocks'. I was met by the Commander, with an anxious look on his face. 'The wife's not at all well, doctor,' he said.

This worried me. He was a nice, sensible old boy who did not take his wife's illnesses too seriously. But he was right. Mrs de Wyrebock looked ghastly. She was sweating profusely, eyes still swollen, and was obviously quite poorly. She was too ill· even to put me in my place. They had motored the day before, in a private ambulance, to have her sinuses X-rayed, so the results could be ready for my visit. It was only their general practitioner they didn't pay, though I did have a sneaking suspicion that they had a private one of these somewhere in London.

I opened the X-ray envelope with trembling hands – it didn't look as if it was going to be my day. The radiologist's report slipped out of the envelope as I was opening it, and before I had time to examine the film. The report was brief – 'X-ray sinuses N.A.D.' Translated, this means 'Nothing abnormal diagnosed.' The clear X-ray plates which I held nervously up to the light confirmed this.

'Well,' said Commander de Wyrebock, 'what is the news, doctor?' I had to play for time. 'Happily the X-rays are clear, Commander,' I said. 'Antibiotics do take a few days to really establish themselves. We'll just carry on with the same treatment. I'll pop in tomorrow. Do give her aspirin if her head is bothering her, and I am sure things will improve in the next twenty-four hours.'

I fled the house, making my way to Janice, wondering what I was going to find, but it was very much the same picture. Her symptoms were worse – temperature, puffy eyes, looking poorly. She, of course, had not had her sinuses X-rayed, but there was obviously no need. There was something going on here that my medical training had not covered. Bill Foulkes looked at death's door; he was complicating the issue by vomiting. I just couldn't think what the hell was wrong with these three, but it certainly wasn't sinusitis.

4

Pork and Means

I was crestfallen when I left my patients and went wearily back to the surgery. What was I going to do? I would have to ask advice from one of my senior partners.

Fortunately Steve was in, sitting smiling behind his desk, with his half-moon gold spectacles. 'Well, Bob, what can we do for you?'

I poured out my story. Whatever could be going on? Steve pointed to a pile of pathology lab. forms on his desk. 'You might be interested to see these blood reports,' he said. I looked, and there were the blood counts of all my three as yet undiagnosed patients – Mrs de Wyrebock, Janice, and Bill Foulkes.

The blood counts all showed one thing: they had more of the type of white blood cells called eosinophils than they should have. Counting the different types of white blood cells in the body can often give a clue to the basic cause of some particular condition. But how did this help? It was getting worse and worse. The only conditions that I knew where you had a raised eosinophil count were in some types of asthmatic chest disease and in parasitic infections like worms.

'What does this mean, Steve?' I asked.

'Well,' said Steve, 'I saw something like this twenty years ago, and I have had five patients probably with the same symptoms as yours, one a nurse sent home from Dilchester Hospital with sinusitis. They all had the same type of blood count.'

Steve was obviously very pleased with himself.

'I also sent some plain blood from my patients and here is the report.'

At last it began to make sense.

The report read, 'Tricinosis larvae seen in the specimen.' This is the parasitic condition you get from eating under-cooked, diseased pork, the pig being the intermediate host for this unpleasant condition.

'But the de Wyrebocks!' I said, 'I can't ever imagine them eating diseased, under-cooked pork. Surely everything they have will be roasted to a turn, and served on a silver platter. Why didn't they all have it? Why just one in each family?'

'In the last epidemic we had like this I carefully questioned everybody. I couldn't understand why a family eating the same meal were not all affected,' said Steve. 'When I looked into it, I found that every patient who contracted the disease finally admitted that at some stage he or she had eaten raw sausage meat.'

'Do they get better?' I asked.

'They are pretty poorly for a few days,' said Steve, 'but they get over it.'

I laughed with relief; the clouds had lifted. I was going to enjoy my visit to Mrs de Wyrebock.

I couldn't get there quickly enough the following day. I walked in, looking serious and thoughtful. Mrs de Wyrebock was looking better than she had been the day before, still not well, but well enough to attack me.

'I don't think you know what is wrong with me, doctor. We would like a second opinion.'

'By all means,' I agreed. 'Who would you like?'

'There is a very good chap in Harley Street we know; we did take the liberty of phoning him and he can come down this evening if needs be.'

'By all means,' I said again. 'I am sure he will be interested in your case. I feel it is quite unique.'

Mrs de Wyrebock perked herself up. She obviously had something rather special.

'I have to ask you one or two more questions,' I said.

'Oh! Couldn't you leave them until the specialist arrives?'

'No, I must establish one or two things before he comes. Have you had any pork recently?'

'Yes, but I can't see what that has got to do with it. Bill Foulkes killed a pig last week. We have had roast pork on two occasions, and I made some sausage meat.'

'Did you have a pinch of the raw sausage meat as you walked through the kitchen?'

Mrs de Wyrebock sat up sharply in bed, blushing, as if she suddenly realised this rather shabby practitioner had either second sight or X-ray eyes.

'Yes, doctor, I did have a pinch when Cook was preparing it – only to see if the seasoning was right.'

'There is the cause of your trouble,' I said. 'You have the parasitic infection that you get from eating uncooked, diseased pork. Your symptoms will disappear in the next few days, and I am sure the specialist will be most interested to see this condition.'

'Err-r-r, I think we are quite satisfied with you, doctor,' rumbled the old Commander. I saw the suspicion of a grin on his face. 'I can't understand our pigs being diseased. We only have the best pedigree stock and they are meticulously looked after. I will look into it.'

'I am afraid the Medical Officer of Health will look into it for you, Commander,' I said. 'These things have to be followed up.'

Janice, who was also a bit better, confessed that she always had a pinch when frying sausage meat as she liked the salty taste. Bill Foulkes took raw sausage meat sandwiches to work. 'They've got a salty bite in the taste,' he explained.

(Bill was the culprit. He was allowed to keep a few pigs on the smallholding he attended himself. When one of his own pigs became a bit sickly he thought it reasonably economic to slaughter his pig and replace it with one from the pedigree herd.)

At the end of my interview with Mrs de Wyrebock, for the first time ever she didn't have very much to say. I packed my bag, and as I left I said, 'I shall need to see you at the surgery next week, Mrs de Wyrebock, to do some further tests.'

'Yes, doctor,' she answered demurely, 'I'll make an appointment.'

I was beginning to win.

Gradually I was settling into the practice. Although I made some mistakes, my partners always backed me up and were a great support and help.

One of the things I found most irritating when out on a home visit, was to be asked if I would pop in next door as they wanted to see me as well. It is not an unreasonable request, but I find that this particular situation irritates doctors out of all proportion. One probably had seven or eight visits still to make, on a tight schedule, to be followed by a surgery. One would go in, seething and reluctant, and with the worst grace treat the extra patient.

After I had blown off steam at coffee one morning about this particular hate of mine, Jack told me how he had come to terms with it. He had been called out to see a child with measles, miles out in the country. Having examined the child he was asked if he would pop in and see the next-door neighbour.

His extra patient was an old man standing by the garden gate, waiting for him. 'I knew you wouldn't mind looking in, doctor,' he said.

Jack, with his hackles at their highest, berated the old man as they walked up to the cottage together, swearing (or so he said) and being generally irritable – he was behind, he had lots of calls, why hadn't the man rung in? The old man walked implacably on, opened the door of the cottage, reached behind the ramshackle settee and pulled out a huge ear trumpet which he screwed into his ear.

'What were you saying, doctor?'

At this point Jack realised that he – and any doctor – had

to be philosophical. The only person he would wear out by a tantrum would be himself.

I asked Jack how he coped with the Burgesses, a family whose hygiene was the poorest of any on our practice list. Not only that, but they kept twenty-two cats and seven dogs, none of which was house-trained or showed any inclination to develop the habit. A few days earlier I had visited the place; the smell almost knocked me over, and it was all I could do not to vomit.

Simple, said Jack. His technique was to walk straight up to the house, open the door, and then walk back to the car to pick up his case. That gave a few minutes for the air to circulate inside the house. He once presented himself in his old A.R.P. gas mask, but the Burgesses thought he was a man from Mars, screamed, and wouldn't let him in.

I still enjoyed my coffee breaks. Steve had a fund of stories about his patients; I never quite believed half of them, but they were part of our morning coffee ritual.

He had one patient, he claimed, who had faithfully produced a new child every year for twelve years, and then suddenly stopped. Steve enquired the reason.

'It's all the fault of Dr Redditch, the local E.N.T. surgeon,' said Mrs Brown. 'You sent me to him, and he fixed me up with a deaf aid. Before I got it, every night when we went to bed my husband used to say "Shall we go to sleep, or what?" And I used to say, "What?"'

Our main surgery was in a converted house about a quarter of a mile from the middle of the town. It had been the home of the town's doctor back in the days when the practice had been a single-handed one. As the town grew, the practice grew, the number of partners increasing over the years to four.

The ground floor of the surgery was taken up with four consulting rooms, four examination rooms, a waiting room from which a reception hatch opened on to the room where the patients' records were kept and the telephone switchboard was situated. We had a small office-cum-laboratory where simple tests could be done, and where a typewriter and tape recorder were kept.

The top two floors were made into flats, one of which was occupied by a retired coal miner and his wife who acted as caretakers. The very top flat, where I lived, was kept by the practice for itinerant locums, assistants and partners such as myself, until such time as they had found their own establishments. It had the chief advantage that Jack and Ivy Bridges, the caretakers, could always take messages at nights and weekends when I was on duty on my own.

We had a full-time reception staff of three. Gladys, a middle-aged spinster and the head of the local Red Cross, went under the title of the Practice Manager. Second-in-command was Mary, who was the wife of the Under Manager at the Colliery. She was quiet and reserved, did all the typing and dealt with the administrative side of the practice. She was a complete contrast to Gladys, who was the least reserved of anyone I have ever met.

Gladys's booming voice dominated the surgery, terrified the patients, and kept us all in step. Far from thinking that she was employed by us, it was Gladys who felt she had four doctors working for her. She spent a great deal of time talking on the telephone to her many friends and colleagues in the Red Cross. One snippet of telephone conversation overheard was Gladys saying she wouldn't have to take on too many commitments over the next couple of months as she had to train a new chap. In spite of her booming, extrovert nature, she had a heart of gold. She got terribly worried if she upset people (which she invariably did), but could always be relied on not to flap in a crisis, and had excellent judgment as to what was urgent and what was not. If Gladys called you for an urgent call, you went.

The final member of the team was Jill, a lovelorn eighteen-year-old who always wore laddered stockings and seemed to be in a perpetual state of distress with yet one more love affair coming to an end. She ran my evening surgeries, usually with tears running down her cheeks. If I asked could I help her, she used

43

to answer, 'No, thank you, doctor. I have just been rather badly let down.'

There was a transient period when she obviously thought I would make a reliable companion, so for two weeks we had immaculate stockings, caked mascara and a plunging neckline that revealed a great deal of her charms. It had a disturbing effect on her work: no lady patient could get past the queue of young men lingering at the hatch asking if she could look up their National Health record number, check their appointments, etc.

Eventually she wilted under pressure. She blushed from ankles to nose when Bill Foulkes, with a loud voice in a packed surgery, said, 'I think I just saw your lungs move, Miss.' Steve, looking whimsically at her cleavage through his gold half-moons asked dryly, didn't she think she might catch a chill?

Although she made no progress with me, she did enrol a fresh batch of unfaithful admirers, and so was soon back to the ladders and the sniffles. The iced gateau that for two weeks had been coming in with my coffee was replaced by digestive biscuits.

I was soon to come under Gladys's command in her capacity as Commandant of the Red Cross. With the added support of Betty, the electrician's wife, who is a trained nurse, she either persuaded or commanded me to become the medical officer to the local Forward Medical·Aid Unit. This is a unit which, in the event of an atomic explosion, is supposed to set up outside the affected town as a sort of casualty clearing station.

We used to rush about with a van and unload ambulances, treat casualties, put on bandages and plaster and give general emergency treatment.

Their enthusiasm at this particular time was due to the fact that the Minister of Health was having a competition to see which was the best Forward Medical Aid Unit in the country. The four first teams were going to have a week-end in London with a grand finale at the Albert Hall, where all would be shaking hands with the great man himself.

The team consisted of a medical officer, a trained nurse and

44

ten auxiliaries. I must say our ten looked a bit long in the tooth, and I was pretty confident that, after our first round, we wouldn't have to bother any more.

We went to our first away competition and to my surprise we won. It was the first time that I had come across a worthy body of people called the Casualties Union. These people spend every Saturday afternoon going round various competitions with bits of Plasticine intestine stuck on their abdominal walls, their faces whitened and plastic blisters stuck to their arms. They are known as Mr Third Degree Burns, Mrs Ruptured Viscer, and Miss Hole in the Chest. They all take it very seriously and most of them were so well drilled and made up that, by the middle of the competition, I got carried away and thought I was treating real casualties.

Having won our first round, the team became even more enthusiastic. Already they could see the lights of London looming.

I was never quite sure what we were supposed to do, but it had become obvious to me that, whatever it was, we seemed to be better at doing it than anybody else. To my great surprise, we won round after round, and the competition final grew nearer and nearer.

We won the regional final, we won the national semi-final, and we were all booked for a trip to London.

Three of our team had never left Tadchester before. Two of them, who had been married over thirty years, had never spent a night away from their husbands. The thought of a night in London – we assumed we would be put up at the best hotel – caused tremendous excitement.

Eventually details of the final came. Far from being put up at Claridges or the Ritz, we were told that accommodation had been found for us at a mental hospital (which I knew only too well from my student days) about twelve miles out of London. This was a big disappointment, but we knew we were going to London, and we were going to the Albert Hall, and the cup was already stuck up in the town hall with our name inscribed on it!

The team got so keen that I wasn't sure whether I was a general practitioner or a full-time F.M.A.U. officer.

We set off for London on a Friday evening. When we arrived at this vast mental hospital (it had 3,500 patients) the girls were put up in the nurses' home, and the hospital secretary and I had to-be put up in the side ward of an observation ward. (The following morning I had to rescue him from a self-locking toilet!)

The next day, with aprons and white coats starched, we set off in our bus for the Albert Hall. We were the first of the four teams in. We represented by far the smallest area, and we were competing against big teams like West London, Rugby and Manchester.

Something ought to have rung a warning bell when they told us the Army was going to assist us.

We were given our instructions by a very brisk military-looking man, who told us that we had to march into the arena as soon as the whistle blew. In the arena I had to report to the Army medical officer in charge. Then we were to take up our action stations.

At this stage, two of the ladies in our team asked if they could spend a penny. Our military man tut-tutted (they were obviously better trained in the Army). He was completely thrown off balance. He was under instructions that we must not be split up as a group, and must be kept under observation until we entered the arena. So, in the charge of an embarrassed corporal, we all marched off to the ladies' toilet. The two ladies' request was obviously infectious as the whole team took this opportunity of relieving their nerves. By the time they had reassembled, with me patiently waiting outside, I was busting to go myself. Whether it was mind over matter or matter over mind, I had to make my own request. There was obviously no sex discrimination here as we were all now marched to the gentlemen's convenience and my team, all trying to look the other way, had to wait until I had finished my ablutions.

At last we were ready. My girls were very nervous. If you

have lived in a small town all your life, to march into the Albert Hall suddenly and make an exhibition of yourself takes some doing. The whistle blew, and we marched into the arena.

There seemed to be scores of Army people and scores of stretchers. I looked round to find the medical officer in charge, and started to do a slow circuit of the floor of the Hall with my team of eleven girls following obediently behind me.

I went round the Hall once, and I could see nobody who seemed to be in charge. Casualties were streaming in, crying, limping, there was blood all over, and I still had nowhere to start work.

I knew I had been round once, because I remembered passing a battle-dressed officer peering into a terrible-looking wound. We circled the Hall again. My girls were getting more and more nervous and the casualties were piling up and bleeding all over the place. We were obviously doing very badly. I passed the officer for a third time.

I could still see nobody who looked remotely as if he were in charge, and seven minutes had gone of the twenty which we were given to treat people.

I eventually came round to the officer again.

'For God's sake,' I exclaimed, 'who is the medical officer in charge?'

'I am,' he said. 'Have you been looking for me?'

I should have expected that the man in charge had even less idea of what to do than I had. By then it was too late. My girls waded into the stacks of casualties that had accumulated, but had hardly coped with any before the whistle went and we all trooped out feeling miserable.

We watched the three other teams come in. The Army medical officer, now alerted, was waiting to greet them and direct them as soon as they came in – except for the third team when again he forgot himself by getting too interested in a case. I knew just how my opposite number felt leading his troop of girls round the floor, but he was stopped after one-and-a-half circuits.

The last team finished. We were all lined up and the results were announced. We were last: our hopes of taking the cup back to Tadchester were crushed.

The winning team from Rugby consisted of a lady doctor, a male staff nurse and ten very fat auxiliaries. They went up to the platform to meet the Minister. They were presented with the cup to tremendous applause. This proved too much for the male staff nurse, who fainted, and had to be supported on either side by two of his stoutest auxiliaries through the whole of the National Anthem.

We trooped off to our bus disconsolately.

'Even if we didn't win,' said Gladys as she mounted the steps, 'we did at least finish on our feet.'

5

Ways of Life and Death

I soon found that routine visiting to the chronic sick and elderly infirm was a very important part of general practice. At first, as a young man itching to try my new medicine, I found it rather tedious, but as time passed I began to realise how important it was: so often the treatment for many conditions was simply to call and see the patient.

The day I qualified, I celebrated in a pub near home. One of the regulars (well into his cups, but still lucid) said, 'So, now you are a doctor! Well, don't forget a doctor's main job is to buck us all up.'

He was dead right. Bucking people up *is* one of the most important things a general practitioner does.

At Tadchester I found I was learning all the time. What seemed insignificant for one person could be a tragedy for another.

One of my regular visits was to an old couple, the Parkers, and the husband's brother. They lived in adjoining farm cottages seven miles out from Tadchester. Brother Jack from next door joined the couple for his meals, but returned to his own cottage to sleep.

Minnie Parker had nursed her diabetic husband for years. He had lost one leg through gangrene, and when I took them over they were battling to save the other – gangrene having appeared in his toe. Normally I would take this as a sign that

49

the other leg was in danger of amputation, but the devoted nursing of Minnie kept the toe gangrene in check for two years. The district nurse used to call twice a day to give him his insulin, but it was Minnie who looked after his toe.

Eventually, when he came to operation, he managed to get away with having just half his foot amputated, enabling him to hobble still with his artificial leg.

They had a most meticulously kept garden and, although all well into their eighties, managed to tend it and more than keep themselves in vegetables and fruit.

The tragedy that struck them was not a medical one. Some sheep broke in through the fence of an adjoining field and ate all the tops off their cabbage and sprout plants. I arrived for my routine call unaware of their disaster, and found them weeping. Heartbroken, they showed me the remaining chewed stumps.

All that was involved, from my point of view, was that there would be three or four dozen cabbages less. Their view of the situation was completely different. This was a tragedy. They couldn't grow their greens for the winter, and travelling to town to buy them was quite out of the question. They could see half a year stretching before them without any vegetables, and there was no way of consoling them.

I had come across this attitude before in elderly people who managed marvellously until some small factor upset their rhythm.

One dear old lady used to give me tea from a beautiful china pot, using her best teaset of delightful china cups. Her house was spotless. She was bright, cheerful, perfectly self-contained and happy.

One day she burnt her finger on the stove, which meant she couldn't lift the teapot, couldn't lift pans off the stove, and couldn't carry on with the same rhythm that she had established.

She died a fortnight later. Although I put 'broncho pneumonia' as the cause of death on her certificate, what she really died of was a burnt finger and an upset life.

50

I used to put aside every second Tuesday of each month for visiting the elderly ladies who lived on the extremities of the practice. The qualification to be included on this round was that they had to be getting on in years and not be fit enough to travel to the surgery to see me. Although none of the ladies that I visited would consider themselves fit enough to come to the surgery, occasionally when I called I found a note saying, 'Out till five o'clock – gone to the chiropodist.' This seemed to be a standard finding – you have to be much fitter to go to see your doctor than to have your toe nails cut.

I liked my old ladies. Two of my favourites were a couple who had lived together since the beginning of World War I – Miss Gill and her companion Miss Booth.

Miss Gill, the elder member of the partnership, had been put to bed in 1916 for some mysterious chest complaint and had never been fit enough to leave it since then. She had spent forty-seven years in bed. Miss Booth had been brought in as her companion in the first year of her illness, and they had lived together since in a small cottage on the main sea road. They had suffered ill health and discomfort with fortitude and dignity for a full forty years before I met them.

Miss Gill used to lie in a bed near the window on a big lace pillow, surrounded by books, and newspaper cuttings from her friends in Canada; she had a mirror arranged so that she could look out of the window and see people passing by.

One would have thought that two ladies who lived at least two-thirds of their lives together in a small cottage, one of them never leaving her bed, would have led a small insular life and gained little from it. On the contrary: they led as successful and contented a life as anyone I ever met. Both these ladies were now in the evening of their lives. Miss Gill had recently celebrated her eightieth birthday. They had a wide circle of friends and a much wider circle with whom they corresponded. My main difficulty was seeing that they did not get overtired with too many visitors.

Miss Gill and Miss Booth were good people by any standards.

51

They were kind; they were what one calls 'practising Christians'. When I came in sometimes and they said, 'We pray every night for you, doctor', somehow I felt ashamed and so very much aware of my own shortcomings.

I eventually realised what pleasures they got from their lives when they showed me some photos of a robin feeding from a tray on Miss Gill's bed. They told me the story of how this robin used to come and perch on the sill outside the window through which Miss Gill looked, waiting for crumbs, how a friendship grew until he was a bold and constant visitor to her room, and how they named him Bobby.

They told me of a particular day when they had a Minister to tea. He put some sponge cake down for Bobby. Bobby, answering the summons of the tapped tray, came in and knocked the sponge cake off the plate – he didn't like cake with no fat in it.

They told me how Bobby brought his mate in and how one day, when he and Mrs Robin were chirping around the room, one of them whistled and a smaller robin, which they thought

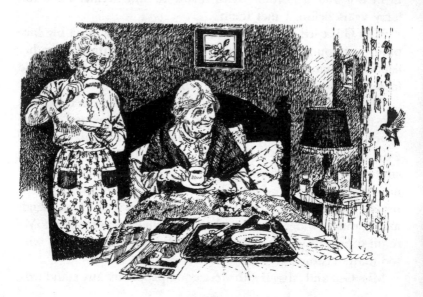

must have been one of the children, came in to join them.

Bobby was their constant visitor for two years. He used to come whenever the tray was banged, and fly around the room. In the winter they put a saucer with food in it by the fire and I imagined them talking to him as they talked to me when I went to see them. They said, 'Do you know, doctor, he even came to say goodbye.'

One day when Bobby came in, it appeared that he had had some blow or injury because he fell four or five times in trying to climb over the window sill. He couldn't stand up, but he managed to eat his crumbs, struggled out of the window, and they never saw him again.

But they still had Bobby's plate to remind them of him.

Miss Gill's and Miss Booth's success story was that their enjoyment had been the company of other people – other people who sought them out in such numbers that they had to be limited on medical grounds – and small incidents like the robin, from which they got such pleasure.

Miss Gill summed it all up one day when she said, 'My difficulty is I see so many people, doctor, because they think I have time to listen.'

Round about Miss Gill's eighty-third birthday the Tadchester Round Table asked if they would like a television set. I wasn't too happy about this; these two ladies had become successfully adjusted to their environment, and now the world, and a very different world from the one they remembered, was going to be brought to their bedside. This could easily upset the whole pattern.

I wondered what their reaction would be if the first programme they saw was a modern play or a cowboy film.

My first visit after delivery of the set dispelled all my fears. I was met by two beaming faces. Miss Gill said, 'Doctor, do you know that for the first time since before the First World War, I have actually taken part in a church service.'

Television was a tremendous success. Sunday with its church services and community hymn singing was their best day. Miss

53

Gill was quite certain that one Sunday the Bishop had nodded to her during the service. Any programme about the Royal Family and people of title came next on their list. Their television took them round castles and cathedrals, introduced them to people of every creed and colour, and showed them some countries and continents as if they were seasoned world travellers. The world they had read and heard about for five decades was suddenly brought into their own little world of four walls and a window.

It never disappointed them, and by some sort of natural selection they never appeared to have tuned into a programme that was objectionable to them.

Miss Gill, whose health had for many years been about as poor as anybody's health could be yet still sustain life, died five months after she received her television set.

I last saw her two days before her death. She lay in bed, her eyes shining and bright, and said, 'We have just seen a most exciting finish to the Lords Test Match, and now I am sitting in the front row of Wimbledon watching the tennis.' Life had never been fuller for her.

It made a deep impression on me and I formed a new respect for television. This wonderful invention had made the last chapter of an eighty-three-year-long life the fullest; it allowed a fine old lady who had been confined to bed for forty-seven years to get up from it, and join in with us for the last few months before she finally left us.

Every other Tuesday I made certain that my last visit of the day was to Reg Dawkins who suffered from a complicated condition called pseudo-muscular hypertrophy of the limb girdle type. Reg was a fit-looking man in his forties who, until he complicated his long-named condition by breaking his hip, used to drive a bus for one of the Tadchester garages. What his condition meant was that there was some lack of nervous connection at waist level so he was left with his legs more or less disconnected from his trunk. Once he was upright, he could walk; once he was sitting, he could drive because he could use his legs; but bending and sitting up unsupported he was no good. Breaking his hip (which had to be operated on) stopped him taking any gainful employment, and he used to sit at home doing odd jobs and cooking from his wheelchair, while his wife, Mary, went out to work.

He was a great wit and I called on'them every other Tuesday to be bucked up rather than to buck them up. I never really gave them any treatment other than an off-work certificate once every three months. Most of their spare time was spent on their hobby of making wine, and every visit I had to sample at least one of the bottles. I used to make it my last call, for a tumbler full of Reg's and Mary's brew laid me out for the evening. My favourite was one called 'Bullous', which was made from wild plums (which I had never seen) – or perhaps it was Reg pulling my leg! It was probably made of old washing-up water.

Mary had three sisters, and I could never fit the right name to the right sister. 'Now Annie is the fat one,' I said. 'No, she isn't,' said Reg, roaring with laughter. 'She's so thin she daren't eat aniseed balls in case she looks pregnant.'·

The longer I stayed in general practice, the more patients I began to know, the more I realised how little I knew. I was learning all the time. I had my own views of what courage and bravery were, but had never examined them closely before.

The first time I was able to recognise sheer courage was when we found that Ben Fellowes had an inoperable growth.

As far as I knew, Ben had led an unobtrusive life. He was an upholsterer. I don't think he had ever been an easy man to work with, but I don't think he had been a terribly difficult one. He lived with his son in a little terraced house Up the Hill.

We had to send him to hospital to be diagnosed.

He accepted hospital life with the aplomb of a countryman, soon settling down to the routine of the ward. He had left things very late before seeking medical advice, and after some investigations it was found that he was far too advanced to be given any help.

Ben somehow got someone to tell him that, not only could

nothing be done, but that he had at the most six months to live. He must have wheedled it out of someone on the pretext of putting his affairs in order, as it was certainly not general policy to tell patients the worst.

When people ask if they are going to die, they ask only to be told they are not. I also didn't accept – and still don't – that a point of hopelessness is ever reached in modern-day medicine, as new cures are found every day and outlooks for certain diseases change overnight.

Past experience had shown me that to be certain of the cause of a disease is to be sometimes wrong. I knew also that, if you take away a man's hope completely, you immediately cut down the amount of time he has left with us.

With this in mind I sent Ben to a deep-ray specialist with a covering note saying that here was a man without any hope, could they possibly do something for him? But again Ben must have done or said something, as back he came with a note saying nothing could in fact be done. This time he even managed to get somebody to tell him that he couldn't live more than three months.

Throughout all this Ben had shown no obvious sign of emotion. He went about in a businesslike manner, putting his affairs in order. He would discuss, openly and unaffectedly, his coming death. He fixed up about his shop, settled his outstanding accounts, and gave me two coronation five-shilling pieces for all the trouble I had taken.

In the first month of the three, Ben went off by train to see and say goodbye to friends, explaining that perhaps he wouldn't be able to get around too well later. He then came back to stay with his son, travelling around with the firm's van or sitting in it quietly by himself behind the row of houses where his son lived, enjoying the last fine days of the summer. From the house Up the Hill there was a fine view of the town, the bridge and the estuary.

I never remember him complaining, and as far as I know he had no faith, creed or philosophy to sustain him. He was always pleased and grateful when I went to see him and never requested anything more than Codeine tablets to relieve whatever anguish he was suffering. He got progressively weaker, and died quietly on the exact day, the end of the three months, predicted as the longest he could live.

I only knew him in this last phase of his life, but I have always felt that he was one of those few men who, spurning hope, had the rare courage to stand up squarely to things as they are. That when he knew the problem without adornments, he said to himself, 'The only thing I have left to do is die. I shall make the best job of it I can.'

Ben was one of many who showed the kind of stoicism and courage I had not met before. Although I thought my patients in Tadchester were different from any elsewhere, I expect that people are much the same everywhere. The life that I had led before I qualified was the unreal one; strange people doing strange things are really the normal people. I looked at everybody that I knew in the area, my partners included, and realised that all of us were a bit offbeat somewhere. I felt (unless I was the odd man out) there must be many things that I did myself that looked strange to other people.

I had done just enough general practice to realise that one had to be aware that there were many things that one didn't understand, and for which there was no real explanation; that patience and observation were the two most important medicines and, although my very specialised knowledge was useful, the most important part of my work was the relationship with my patients and our understanding of each other.

6

Miraculous Draughts

I had been in the practice about six months when, one night, Kevin and Janice Bird rang to say, 'Tonight we are going to initiate you into Seine net fishing. You can bring Eric along if you like. Frank's taking his net out and is looking for a new crew.'

Frank Squires was the land surveyor for the County Council and lived with his wife way out on the estuary. It was like a small zoo, with goats, chickens, geese, ducks, cats, dogs, rabbits, and strange species of birds I was never able to identify. He depended on his salary for his living, but his life was the open air, the country, and the sea.

He had one-and-a-half acres of land which he ran like a small-holding. He sailed, fished, and was the leader of this mysterious clique that I had heard of, called 'Seine Fishers' who, at low tide, trailed their nets along the two beaches of Sanford-on-Sea. There were tales of huge catches and stormy seas. It all sounded a bit improbable.

'Bring your rugger shorts,' said Kevin, 'as many old jumpers and shirts as you have got, and something to wear on your feet.'

It seemed to me, if we were going to be wading about in the sea, a pair of bathing trunks would have been enough, but I took his advice and took a whole pile of old clothes with me.

We assembled on the beach that night at about ten o'clock.

When the tide is out at Sanford there is plenty of beach – it goes out for over a mile.

There was Frank, obviously in command, in a pair of shorts, with a short oilskin jacket, a piece of rope tied firmly round his middle, and an old felt hat jammed on his head.

'Come on, Dr Bob. Get your gear.'

'Won't bathing trunks be enough?' I asked.

'No,' said Frank, 'you will freeze to death if you don't keep yourself covered.'

There were eight of us in all – Janice and Kevin, Eric and myself, Frank and his wife Primrose, Joe Church – a bearded schoolmaster – and his wife Lee.

We marched out towards the sea, with Joe and Frank carrying a couple of poles on their shoulders, around which was wound a length of nylon net. Walking behind, the ladies pulled a little sledge which was really a box on two runners. The sledge was there, hopefully, to carry the fish.

We arrived at the water's edge and separated the two poles to which the net was attached. The net was sixty yards of nylon net, about six feet in depth, and each of the poles had two rope traces. These were attached to the middle of the pole. The pole was held upright in the water by the pole carrier. One or two people in front tugged and pulled the lengths of rope traces and helped the pole tow the net along during the trawling.

'You can come on the outer staff with me,' said Frank, 'and Eric can go on the inner with Joe.'

Frank then slipped the pole diagonally across his chest, Kevin and I took a trace rope each and walked off into the sea in front of him. Although the sea struck cold at first, our protective clothing kept the wind out and we soon warmed up.

The beach shelved gradually and we must have walked out two hundred yards before the water had reached chest height. There was a little bit of surf and as we walked we were continually jumping up to ride the waves, or ducking and letting them splash over us.

It was exhilarating, and great fun.

'Right,' shouted Frank when the water was up to our armpits, 'now we start work.'

Kevin and I tightened the trace ropes round our shoulders and started to tug at the staff that Frank was holding, walking along parallel to the beach, every few minutes either being lifted or covered by waves, pulling ourselves up on the ropes, laughing and spluttering.

The waves were fluorescent in the partial moonlight, and as I looked back I could see that Joe, with Eric tugging in front of him, had joined us in a parallel course to the beach. They were about twenty yards behind us and forty yards in, and the net was travelling along parallel to the beach like a letter 'J', the long arm of the 'J' being the outer one.

Frank's face glowed like an isolated skull with the fluorescent sheen from the water, the rest of his silhouette of black clothes being lost in the darkness.

We tugged and pulled for about twenty-five minutes. By now I certainly wasn't cold. I could have even been sweating under my wet clothes.

'Right,' said Frank. 'Let's have a draught.'

We swung round, going directly up the beach. Kevin's pole kept moving towards us until they were about ten yards away, then with the whole net taut, we marched side by side towards the beach, the net in a long thin 'U' streaming behind us.

I couldn't see that we had caught anything. I could make out the floats on the top of the net, bobbing behind us, but no sign of splashing fish, or signs of the huge hauls that I had heard about.

We steadily got nearer the beach, until the water came down to our mid-calves, but still nothing to see in the back of the net. Then we were on the sand, marching slowly up the beach, the net getting heavier all the time. Looking back, I saw a flash of white at the base of the 'U' of the net, and as we got into shallower water – to my excitement – I could see several splashes.

I dropped my rope to rush back to see the haul. I picked it up again when Frank bellowed, 'Keep pulling you stupid bugger! You will lose the catch! Keep pulling!'

We pulled on until the net was on dry sand, and then rushed back. I could see thrashing bodies of white in the base of the 'U' that now came almost to a point on the dry sand.

'Lights!' shouted Frank, and the girls came rushing up with torches, tugging their box behind them.

The bottom and top ropes of the net were together encasing the fish. When these were opened, I could see four flat fish and three round fish.

'Quick! Give me the trout!' shouted Frank, snatching up one of the round fish and shoving it under his jumper. 'We don't want to be caught with this.'

Frank identified the rest of the catch – two bass, three dabs and one sole.

The fish he had shoved under his jumper was a sea trout. Although we were fishing off a sandy beach that is packed with holiday makers in the summer, it still came under the River Authority, which did not allow game fish (which included sea trout) to be taken from the sea. Frank had twice been caught by water bailiffs and was due to lose his net if caught again.

I thought we had finished for the night, but I was wrong. This was just the beginning.

We made six more draughts, covering at least two miles of beach, and caught about thirty fish. On only two of the draughts did the net come out of the sea empty. The catch included slimy skate, whose little eyes appeared to be looking up straight at you; a chad, a sort of king herring that I had never heard of before; some more bass, which the locals prized more than salmon or sea trout; some mullet, which the rest turned their noses up at as they reckoned these were the scavengers of the sea; and two more small sea trout which were immediately hidden in the pockets of Joe's oilskin.

The rest of the catch was dumped into the box, now full to the brim with fish. We trudged back to the cars parked in the sandhills, now two miles away, where the road goes down to the beach.

The journey seemed endless. We had to carry the heavy, sodden net, which seemed to weigh a ton. My legs were getting cold as the wind swept along the beach. It had been much warmer in the water.

At last we got back to the cars, had a brisk rub down, and put on dry clothes.

I felt like a king.

Frank got a primus stove going, and we soon had hot coffee and sandwiches. I had not felt so fit in years.

The catch was divided evenly in what I understood was the traditional Seine-netting way of doing it. Frank stood with his back to the five piles of fish, and (unseen) Joe, behind him, would point to one and ask, 'Whose is this?' Frank would shout 'Eric' or 'Joe' till we all had a name to a pile and rushed up to see what our particular share was.

My share was a bass, one of the small sea trout, two dabs and a mullet. I had never had so much fish on my hands before and wondered what I was going to do with it.

'Now,' said Frank, 'don't forget you must clean your fish before you go to bed, otherwise it will be no use to anyone.'

Eric dropped me off at the surgery and I heaved my parcel of fish into the sink behind the dispensary, got an old scalpel from the cupboard, and tried to remember my days as a first-year medical student when the nearest I got to being a surgeon was operating on a dogfish. They say you really have to start at the beginning to practise medicine.

Cleaning the fish gave me some surprises. They were all quite different. The sea trout was almost spotless and aristocratic, and cleaned easily; the mullet was like a dirty old tramp, and filthy intestines came from it. I did not fancy it. The bass was halfway between both worlds – middle class – and the flat fish took very little cleaning.

I gutted them, washed them, put them in a polythene bag and put them in the fridge.

I was desperately tired by now and looked up at the surgery clock. My God! It was a quarter to four.

I shovelled all the offal from the fish into the dispensary pedal bin, washed up as best I could, then crept up to my flat, threw myself on the bed and went to sleep. I had a free morning the following day, thank goodness.

I woke up about ten and made myself a cup of tea. I was out of condition, not having taken much exercise since I had come to Tadchester, and was feeling a few muscles that I had not felt before.

I must have dozed off. There was Gladys banging on the door, and it was a quarter to two.

'Come on, Dr Bob, you have a surgery in ten minutes! It is a wonder there is a surgery here at all today – the whole place stinks like a fish shop. Wait till Dr Maxwell gets hold of you! He went to the refrigerator to get some penicillin and was almost buried by an avalanche of fish. You have a big surgery this afternoon and a medical afterwards, so look lively.'

I hurriedly dressed and shaved and went down. Gladys was right; it was a big surgery. It seemed to go on for ever. I could hardly keep my eyes open, and my muscles felt like knots. But at last I finished.

Gladys bustled in, with a cup of tea. She had a peculiar grin on her face when she said, 'I thought you might like a bit of refreshment before your medical, doctor. I think it is going to be a long and difficult one.'

I was a little puzzled but, in my exhausted state, did not take too much notice. I rang the bell for the medical examination, and in walked Gwendoline Jacobs, our beauty queen. Oh, God! This was all I needed. She was certainly not a girl to be deterred.

She was wearing a black plastic raincoat, fishnet stockings, and long black boots. As she took off her coat I noticed that if her skirt had been any shorter it would have started just under her arms. The plunge of her neckline started somewhere near her knees.

'Shall I get undressed, doctor?' she said.

63

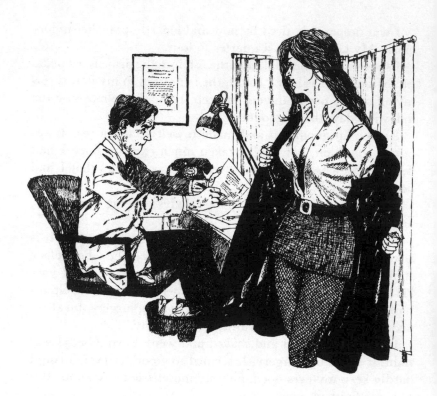

'No. Hang on, Gwendoline,' I said. 'I have a lot of questions to ask you first.'

I sat down and went laboriously through all the medical questions – date of mother's death, age of father if living, brothers, sisters, previous medical history, regularity of periods, etc., with Gwendoline looking straight into my eyes, leaning over the desk as if she were trying to eat me. She signed my record of questions and answers as being correct, then, with her eyes lit up – 'Now, doctor?'

'Yes,' I said, resignedly. 'Pop behind the screen and get undressed. You will find a sheet on the couch.'

She was off in a flash.

I couldn't help liking Gwendoline. There was something quite charming about her open sexuality.

She lay on the couch with the white sheet tucked firmly under her chin.

I took her pulse and blood pressure without disturbing her enveloping shroud. I was putting off the time when the surprises underneath it would be revealed to me.

'Now, I would like to have a look at your chest.'

She smiled in anticipation and sat bolt upright. Her breasts were supported in the same sort of material as her stockings. I must say it enhanced their silhouette.

'You will have to take your brassière off, Gwendoline,' I said.

'Oh! If you could just help me, doctor. It has a difficult clip at the back.'

She sat up, breasts bulging out of their restraining nets, and shoulders arched. I did a retreating battle, trying to unclip her bra as she tried to lean back on me.

She lay back, naked from the waist up, eyes half closed, as if in a dream. I put my hand on her upper abdomen. She let out a contented 'Ah!' and two deep purple nipples shot up like fountain pen caps with such speed that it made me jump back on my heels.

I hastily withdrew my hand, then listened to her chest, making sure it was only my stethoscope that touched her. I looked down her throat and into her ears while Gwendoline purred and writhed gently with delight or passion, but she still kept a twinkle in her eye.

'I have finished with the top half now,' I said. 'You can dress up there and we will tackle the other half.'

She struggled into her bra and blouse disappointedly, then slowly slid the sheet down to expose a sun-tanned stomach and the smallest pair of bikini pants that I have ever seen. Boldly printed on the front of them were the words, 'COULDN'T WE TALK THIS OVER?'

I had the greatest difficulty in stopping myself laughing.

Gwendoline looked up. 'Oh! I do apologise, doctor, I had forgotten I'd got these silly old things on.'

To Gwendoline's squirms of delight I palpated her stomach, tested her reflexes, and eventually finished my examination.

'That's all, Gwendoline,' I said. 'Thank you. You can get dressed now.'

'Is there nothing else, doctor? How do you know I am all right internally? Shouldn't that be checked?'

By now I was having great difficulty in preventing myself bursting out laughing. It was painful holding my sides in. I took up the examination form, pretending to study it closely, and said, 'No, thank you Gwendoline, I have carried out all the tests that they asked me to.'

Gwendoline ruefully started putting her clothes on as I retired back to my desk. I was determined to win this battle.

She came round from behind the screen, adjusting her skimpy clothing.

'Oh! There is just one more thing, Gwendoline,' I said. Her eyes lit up. 'Could you leave a specimen of urine with Gladys on your way out.'

She gave me a withering look, but she was not beaten yet. She put her hand in her handbag, shoved a ticket on my desk and said, 'There is a spare ticket for the Carnival Ball, doctor. I said that I knew you would come and present the prizes.'

She shot out of the door before I had time to give it back to her.

Gladys came in disdainfully. 'It must have been a complicated medical, doctor, for you to take so long, but I expect you can't skimp anything on someone so young. I think it's about time you found yourself a Mrs Clifford, or one of these bright young things is going to nab you.'

With Gladys and Gwendoline gone I checked through the notes of the people I had seen in the afternoon surgery. One or two of them would need follow-up visits, and three had to go for back X-rays of one sort or another.

Backache, I found, was an extremely common condition in general practice. It has replaced grandmother's funeral as a reason for a day off, and more of the most miraculous cures I saw were achieved by the settlement of compensation claims for injuries received at work. I would see a patient bent double, going round the tribunals and being assessed for his degree of disability. The next day I would see the same man again, upright, pitching hay or carrying hundredweight sacks of potatoes. It was not that he had had some miracle drug or miracle cure – it just meant his compensation claim for backache had been settled.

Backache cases were always springing surprises on me. Sometime previously, when Jack Dawson came complaining, I thought it must be in some way connected with his work at Thudrock Colliery.

He was a huge man, six foot three, eighteen stone, and famous for his boxing ability. He had, some years back, been a full-time pro, but now only came into his own the autumn week that the travelling fair visited Tadchester. He would appear on the first day, knock out all the new professionals in the boxing booth, then be employed by the booth, taking on all-comers for the remainder of the week. Any prize money he won would have gone on beer before the end of the night, but he was a goodtempered, amiable giant, slow to anger, and just the man to have on your side if there was trouble brewing. His presence alone was enough to dispel any thought of aggression by opponents.

Jack had a severe pain in the lower back, with pain going down the leg – obviously sciatica with a spinal nerve being trapped. He could hardly move.

I thought, with his strength and size, he must be at least a full-blown collier, thrashing away at the coal face with a pick all day, but not so. He actually worked in the pit-bottom office as a time-keeper's clerk, supplementing his income by taking betting slips for the local bookies.

I sent him home to bed with some pain killers, and visited him on his smallholding the next day. He lived with his wife, mother and daughter in a delightful thatched cottage in about four acres where he kept a few pigs and poultry. Sitting by the steps of the cottage when I arrived was an old lady (presumably

67

his mother) who was just finishing off peeling a whole bucket of potatoes.

'Are you having a party, Mrs Dawson?' I asked.

'Oh! No,' she replied. 'We do a bucketful of these every day. This is my job.'

Jack was not in bed as directed – perhaps he had just come for a ticket after all. Eventually I found him in one of the poultry houses, where he greeted me with a, 'Good morning, doctor. I thought I'd work off a bit of the stiffness.'

As he was speaking to me, he continued to wring the neck of a poor chicken which was obviously going to accompany the waiting half hundredweight of peeled potatoes.

He wrung the bird's neck with no more qualms than he would have swatted a fly. There were obviously no emotional ties between him and this chicken.

'Well, what about this back, Jack?' I asked. 'Is it better, or what?'

'It is much better, doctor,' he said, 'but not quite right for work. I think it is my part-time job that's the cause of it. I think I'll have to give it up.'

I knew Jack worked down the pit. I knew he was a bookies' runner. I knew he farmed his smallholding. His appearances at the fair were famous, and I felt sure that he did a bit of poaching with salmon nets. What else could he be doing as a part-time job?

'I keep rather quiet about it,' said Jack. 'They say at the place we shouldn't talk too much about it. I am sometimes a relief hangman.'

Now I understood about the chicken.

I was then treated to a half-hour lecture on the art of hanging, of how the weights put an extra strain on your back. Apparently the ropes have to be tested with the equivalent weight of the intended victim. This means a whole lot of lifting of sandbags, up to a hundredweight, with the chance that if you had got your calculations wrong they could fall on top of you. I couldn't take it in. I was completely bemused by it all.

'If you could give me a certificate, doctor,' he said, 'I could send it to the Home Office. I really don't think I should do hanging any more. I can't let this back interfere with my normal work. I have a lot of people depending on me. I don't do hangings very often, but if they are going to interfere with my real livelihood, I'll call it a day.'

My certificate to excuse Jack his hanging duties apparently cured his back. He never came complaining of it again. I don't know whether they compensated him for his loss of earnings, but I did get a couple of badly plucked chickens left at the surgery by him soon after he had hung up his rope.

7

All in the Mind

The psychiatric services available in Tadchester were very limited. Once a week a consultant from the mental hospital outside Winchcombe used to hold an outpatients' clinic in this hospital: half of his time he would spend interviewing patients and the other half giving courses of E.C.T. (electro convulsive therapy) to patients under treatment.

I have never got on terribly well with psychiatrists: I often find it difficult to distinguish them from their patients. No man should spend all his time doing psychiatry.

Most of general practice is psychiatry of one sort or another, but you are seeing other patients with organic illnesses who help to maintain a balance. I was never sure how helpful psychiatric referral was to my patients and sometimes tossed up whether I should send a patient in trouble for a psychiatric consultation or for a course of physiotherapy. There seemed little to choose between the results.

Whatever treatment patients with psychiatric illnesses were having and whatever the psychiatrist thought he was doing, there was no doubt that we in general practice carried the brunt of most cases.

Mr Shannon, the local chief inspector of taxes, died suddenly and unexpectedly of a coronary in his office. He and his wife had been very happily married. She was completely overwhelmed by her tragedy and just could not cope. She became disorientated and I had to visit her daily, giving what support I could, together with various medications, to help take the edge off her fears and anxieties. She was an intelligent, well-balanced woman who just could not manage the situation she found herself in.

I seemed to be making little progress with her so I asked for a psychiatric opinion. I had a very long letter back from the psychiatrist telling me what I already knew, suggesting similar medication to that which I was giving, and saying he would see Mrs Shannon again in a month's time.

Mrs Shannon tried the psychiatrist's medication but preferred mine. She showed some small improvement in that, instead of my making daily visits to her house, she made daily visits to the surgery. This, initially, was a tremendous effort for her but a sign of a real step forward.

After a month she was seen again by the psychiatrist who, in a ten-minute interview, managed to upset her on several counts. He was impressed that she was improving and decided that she could wait two months until her next interview with him.

Mrs Shannon still visited me nearly every day. My main treatment was constantly to reassure and encourage her, repeatedly telling her that time to some extent would heal and that things would improve. Slowly she began to adjust and get back into a normal pattern of life. I encouraged her to find some sort of work and eventually she found a part-time job in Mr Southern's solicitor's office.

As arranged, she saw the psychiatrist after a two-month interval. He wrote me a short note saying that 'his' treatment had seemed effective in this case and he had discharged Mrs Shannon from his outpatients' clinic. 'Bully for him,' I thought.

I continued to see Mrs Shannon at decreasing intervals – three times a week, twice a week, then once a week, till we arrived at a situation where she popped in for a chat once a month to report that all was going well. It was a full two years before she felt there was no need to come and be consoled about her grief any more.

Assisting the psychiatrist was a marvellous breed of men called Mental Welfare Officers. They were men usually in or around their forties who had been trained as nurses and mental nurses, and were the people to call on when you were in real trouble with psychiatric emergencies. I valued their services at least as much as the psychiatrist's.

Jack Turner had a long history of psychiatric disturbances. When he became ill, he became very violent and aggressive and, as he weighed eighteen stone, he was very difficult to cope with. It was usually the police who rang us when Jack went on one of his destructive campaigns. We would arrive at the house to find the police prudently waiting outside, listening to the sounds of smashing glass and furniture from within. Then we would all charge in as a body and try to overpower him long enough for me to get a sedative injection into him. Once he was reasonably quiet he was put into a strait-jacket and taken off to hospital.

One of the most bizarre psychiatric emergencies I was called to was on a country farm just beyond the edge of our practice area A woman patient of mine was on leave from Winchcombe Mental Hospital and had come out to impose herself on two ladies who lived as man and wife in this isolated farmstead. They had met while having psychiatric treatment, and this was one of those love triangles between three ladies that I could never quite understand.

My patient, on arriving at the farmhouse and finding that neither of the residents would respond to her amours, tried to form a close relationship with a boxer dog. The two resident ladies, at their wits' end, managed to get her out of the house and lock her in a shed with one of the cows, leaving her to get on with it. It was all very sad. They were all young, attractive women. I wondered what paths had led them to this present situation.

Here again the Mental Welfare Officer and I had a fighting

scramble to slam in the sedative injection and put a strait-jacket on and get the poor disturbed girl off to hospital.

I found that as well as having to be at least a half-time amateur psychiatrist, I was keeping open a twenty-four-hour consultation service. It appeared I was even more reassuring on the phone than I was in the flesh. People used to ring at all hours with the most unusual worries. A common complaint was that, while bathing, they had found a little hard lump just at the bottom of their breastbone. Was it cancer? Of course it wasn't. We all have a little hard lump there. It is made of cartilage and it is called our xiphisternum. It was surprising the number of people who spent sleepless nights after finding it.

The bath was a great place for the discovery of moles, warts, lumps, and – just very occasionally – something of significance like a lump in the breast.

The medical problems I could cope with: it was the non-medical ones that took up most of my time. I was asked advice on house purchase, car purchase, the best time of the year to get married, and several times consulted about the health of various animals – dogs, cats, and once even a cow that was in labour.

Only once do I remember not coming up with some sort of answer. At ten o'clock one night I was rung by an anxious mother. Her son had won a talent contest for singing at the holiday camp from which they had just returned. Did I think he ought to cut a record? I had been up the whole of the previous night and had risked having a bath and getting into bed at eight o'clock. I couldn't give an answer – but nearly suggested that she cut his throat.

I had to explain to some people that running out of the Pill at eleven o'clock at night was not an emergency, and that you should ring up for advice before 10.45 p.m. to ask whether you are likely to get sunburnt in Majorca or not. Also, even more gently, I had to persuade people that one o'clock in the morning was not the time to seek advice about a fortnight's constipation.

The best treatment for so many conditions is reassurance: the negative result of an investigation often gives relief from actual pain as well as worry. I have seen intelligent, well-balanced people genuinely short of breath with crippling chest pains and in a mental torment waiting for their chest X-ray results. As soon as they knew their chest X-ray was clear, they lost all their symptoms and became one hundred per cent fit again.

Steve helped greatly in managing this sort of problem. He was kind, wise, and philosophical.

'Bob,' he said, 'one of our most important jobs is saving people's faces with themselves. You have to try and judge when you think a patient is about to break down and, by anticipating it, stop it happening. You will have patients coming to you, men and women, over-tired, over-anxious, exhausted and worried, wanting to be told what to do. Somehow you have to give them direction, and make them think that they have chosen this direction themselves.

'As a doctor you carry a certain authority. The patient believes this, and the people they are in contact with believe it too. If they go out armed with the message "the doctor says I must do this" or "the doctor says I mustn't do that", people will take notice.

'You will have to use your judgment about when you intervene in people's lives. If you find someone at the end of their tether, you may have to step in and direct them for a time, such as insisting that they go off work with a sick note for a spell, giving a specific reason, such as nervous exhaustion or a viral infection, for their spell off work. Whatever reason you give must save their pride, or they will otherwise take it as confirmation of their inadequacy.

'You may have to be firm with your direction, threatening them that if they don't take your advice, then they are in danger of cracking up. So often you will find they are hardly able to hide their relief on being directed. It is a bit like playing God, but providing you are not presumptuous or conceited about it, then it is a responsibility you have to take. This is general practice.

'There is a story,' he said with a smile, 'of an Archbishop

74

who died and went to heaven. He found he had to join a queue at the pearly gates, to be let in by St Peter. The Archbishop got irritated standing in this long queue, walked up to St Peter and said, "I am the Archbishop. Surely I don't have to wait in the queue like other men?" St Peter replied, "All men are equal here. I am afraid you will have to wait your turn." Standing disgruntled in the queue, the Archbishop noticed an old whiskered man on a bicycle, with a case strapped on the back, cycle the full length of the queue, knock on the gates, and go straight in. The Archbishop rushed up indignantly to St Peter and said, "I thought all men were equal here. How was it that old man could jump to the head of the queue and get in? Why should he be favoured?" "Oh," said St Peter, "that's God Himself; occasionally he likes to go back down to earth and play doctor." '

In spite of all the available medical services, psychiatric and general, many people continue to lead offbeat lives of their own. It is impossible to collect statistics of people who hide behind doors, because normally you never see them. As a general practitioner, with access to most homes, you find situations that normally never see the light of day.

One bank clerk, who to all outward appearances led a fairly normal life, I found spent most of his off-duty hours in a sort of blanket tent underneath the dining-room table. It was the only place he felt really safe in. As he managed most of his life pretty well, one couldn't interfere. I learnt later that several of his family had been killed in an air raid during the war: he had survived, protected by an old billiard table that he had been sleeping under.

Quite a number of people felt that other people were shining rays at them, or that there were men hiding in the television set, watching them. They would listen patiently to all your reassurances and then slip straight back into their little fantasy world.

Tadchester had its share of people with phobias. The most common were the agoraphobics – people who were terrified of wide open spaces. But there are phobias – i.e. irrational, illogical fears – about everything. I found, for example, that one girl's insomnia and bad school report were due to a bus phobia. She was literally terrified of being in or anywhere near a bus. She didn't know why, and there was no obvious reason for her fear.

I found these patients (particularly the children) most difficult to treat. It took a tremendous time of patient reassurance and encouragement to help them find the reserves of courage to face up to, and conquer, their fears.

There is so much that we don't know about mental illness and mental breakdown and I feel we are just at the beginning of our knowledge and could well not be pursuing the right lines of investigation. It is possible that there could be as much mental and psychiatric background to an acute appendicitis case as there is in some other poor disturbed patient whom we write off as being queer.

There are a few disturbed people who literally suffer the agonies of the damned, and who can be helped very little. Ron Towle was one.

Ron's was the most time-consuming psychiatric disorder that I ever had to cope with. More than most patients, he made me feel that psychiatric illness is just as real, and probably as organic, as pneumonia, pleurisy and even heart disease.

I saw him more than I saw any other patient over a period of five or six years. Sometimes he would make an appointment to see me: more often he would hang about in the surgery trying to catch me after the last patient, when he knew that I would have no excuse to cut short my time with him.

He was a short, prematurely grey man in his late forties, dressed shabbily in an old raincoat. His general appearance was unkempt, with frayed collars and cuffs and scruffy shoes. He had come from a good family, been away to boarding school, and was not without money. He was a sort of general dealer, buying and selling cattle, land, and turning his hand to sell anything that might make a profit. He drove round Tadchester in an old Austin Seven which he kept meticulously.

His main worries he related to his business deals. I would see him through one deal, supporting him through the traumas, and he would collect his money (most often he made a profit). Ten days later he would be walking up and down inside my consulting room, beating his chest and saying what a fool he had been, how he had got involved in another deal, he would lose all his money, people were taking advantage of him ... and so we would go on.

He was always in a terrible torment with himself, coming up with new symptoms. He had been many times admitted to the mental hospital, he had had every sort of psychiatric treatment, but it never seemed to lessen the torment. He would say, 'There is something terrible happening in my head, and you just don't understand. Why doesn't someone do something about it?'

I grew quite fond of him and sympathised with his turmoils. Some days he was better and would come in and chat. He was well educated, widely read, and was conversant with all the main topics of the day. He would talk for hours, given a chance. He had quite an infectious grin, but most days he would be beating his chest in despair, despairing about his attire, about his accommodation, about how far he had come down in life. He would eat up as much listening time as I was prepared to give him.

He lived in a small house in Park Lane, outside the park, four doors away from the prim Sophie and Elsie Emmerson. Somehow he was unable to join in society and make friends and communicate with people normally. He shaped his life in isolation around his business deals. In the same way that they destroyed him, they were also the things that kept him going. Our standing joke, when he came in, was, 'Well, Ron, have you bought the Eiffel Tower yet?'

Sometimes his business deals were out of town, and he would go off in his little car and come back chest beating, again moaning about some new venture he had got involved in: it was going to be his ruin, he was going to lose all the little money he had.

At his worst he became very disturbed. If I wasn't at hand

to settle him down, most often he would have to be forcibly admitted to the mental hospital.

Once, I went away for a weekend, after having seen Ron nearly every day for three months. He had a breakdown, was admitted to hospital for three days, then came storming in to the surgery accusing me of not being there when he needed me. I had let him down.

For one short period of a few weeks he seemed fine and well-balanced. He had been off to London to see some offbeat medical therapist whose consulting room was the back parlour of a council house in Clapham. Ron was cured. For those few weeks, whatever magic this young man from Clapham had performed on him seemed to work.

Ron's great desire was to be normal, to be accepted, to be married, but he never ever made it. He was on various medications, some of which seemed to help him, some of which obviously upset him. There seemed to be no area that we had not explored where he could be given special help for his torment. Ron really knew that nobody could help his particular case, and he was incapable of helping himself.

One day, as was always likely, he was found dead in his house. He had taken an overdose of tablets, whether by accident or design we will never know. I think it was by accident because he had always clung tenaciously to life, hoping that things would improve.

I feel that, as research progresses, help one day for the small group like Ron will be found, that their disturbance will have some chemical or physiological background. There was a time when you knew that if you had sugar diabetes or pernicious anaemia, there was no known cure. Nowadays people with these complaints can look forward to a normal and full life-span with small inconveniences of injections and diet. I think the time will come when poor unfortunates like Ron will be able to share these same expectations.

When I was a medical student and we were visiting mental hospitals, we had a patient pointed out to us who always claimed that he was tuned in to the BBC Light Programme. It was a great joke, but years later, I have often wondered whether in fact he was right. I found in general practice that so many problems had no answer – it was a matter of continual support and keeping people going, with not always a happy ending.

8

Curious Cures

Not long after I had given Gwendoline Jacobs her medical examination I found that things started to happen to me for which I couldn't find an explanation.

One night I had to swap surgery because Janice and Kevin Bird had asked me to a dinner party. I hadn't told anybody except Jill, my evening receptionist, about my change of plan, but at least half the patients who came on the wrong night knew about the change already.

On one or two calls in the country I would be flagged down by patients who would say, 'I heard you were coming this way, doctor, could you call in on me on your way back?' Something really strange was happening.

It was when I was taking complicated directions from a patient at Sanford-on-Sea about how to get there that my problem was solved – or that my problem really began. In the middle of our conversation a voice chipped in: 'You would be much better turning right by the gasworks, doctor, and going along the sea road.'

The voice was unmistakable. It was Gwendoline. I had forgotten that she worked on the telephone exchange. God, how many other of my conversations had she listened in to?

From then on Gwendoline haunted me. I was almost terrified

to pick up the phone. If she were taking my call I had a terrible time getting through her chit chat to actually get a number. She was always pressing me to go to parties, picnics or barbecues, and whenever I was asking for directions to outlandish places it always became a three-part conversation.

The trouble was she was sometimes useful – almost too useful. She would hang on to calls, knowing I was out, and save them till I got back. She became an unofficial receptionist, and in fact asked during one of our many conversations whether I would consider her for a job at the surgery if one ever became vacant, as she was very good on the phone.

I noticed that whenever Marjorie de Wyrebock phoned me (and her phone calls had begun to increase in number) that we were always getting cut off. Sometimes a very high-pitched, falsetto voice which was obviously Gwendoline's in disguise, would say 'So sawry. There seems to be a fault on the line.'

I could think of no answer to this particular problem. I daren't mention it to my partners – they would have laughed at me. If the phone rang when we were all having coffee together, I froze and never volunteered to pick it up. I couldn't really complain to the Post Office that one of their telephonists was being too helpful.

My haunting by Gwendoline went on for about two months. I was getting to a point of near despair when, in the middle of one evening surgery, I saw that one of the names on the patients' appointments list was Mrs Daphne Jennings, the telephone supervisor. I wondered could I use her to frighten Gwendoline off?

When Mrs Jennings came through the door, I saw to it that I was on the phone to Kevin. When Kevin answered the phone I started to ask him the most complicated directions to a place fifteen miles along the coast. I knew this was a bait that Gwendoline couldn't refuse. Once I had asked Kevin the question, I looked down at my watch and said, 'Help! I have an appointment to see Dr Maxwell. I wonder, Mrs Jennings, if you would mind taking these directions from Mr Bird?'

I gave Mrs Jennings the phone, dashed out of the room, and waited. Would my dastardly plot work?

I stayed out for ten minutes and then came back into the room. Mrs Jennings was like a beetroot, and hardly able to contain herself.

'How often does that girl interrupt telephone conversations?' she asked.

'Oh, I think she only tries to be helpful,' I said.

'We'll see about her being helpful tomorrow morning,' said Mrs Jennings.

That was the last I heard on the telephone from Gwendoline Jacobs.

I gathered she couldn't be sacked from the Post Office: as well as being the Carnival Queen, she was Miss Post Office for that year. However, she was demoted from the switchboard and sent to sort letters in the corrugated-iron shed that served for this purpose behind the main Post Office.

With Gwendoline off the phone, Marjorie de Wyrebock had no difficulty in getting through to me. She seemed to be able to find an excuse to ring me most days. It was either an invitation to a hunt ball or to ask why didn't I take riding lessons? She apologised for being the initial cause of my riding accident, and as she ran the local livery stables and was quite a good horsewoman (to judge by the size of her buttocks and thighs, she had been at it for many years) she would be my obvious instructor. I sometimes almost wished that Gwendoline was back jamming the calls again.

About this time I started to build up a regular eccentric clientele that was offbeat even for Tadchester. For some reason, they all turned up at my Wednesday evening surgery, over which Jill presided, surrounded by her usual ring of admirers asking for acne tablets.

There was Miss Bessie Oldthorpe from the sweetshop – she weighed 18 stone 3 pounds. I might have been forgiven for thinking she wanted to lose weight, but no! If her weight ever fell below 18 stone 1 pound, she thought she had a cancer, and I had great difficulty in reassuring her. She went about in mortal fear until she had regained the missing two pounds.

The only time she did lose weight was when – on very shaky grounds – she thought she might be pregnant. She lost two stones in three weeks, worrying, until Nature reassured her. Then she lost almost another two in trying to regain the weight she'd lost, to prove she hadn't got a cancer.

Next came Harry Jones. One must admit that Harry was a little simple. He always came in with the same symptom – he thought people knocked him out when he wasn't looking. He never had any bruises or marks, neither did he remember it happening; but as he logically argued, 'If someone knocks me out from behind when I'm not looking, how would I know?' And, of course, he was right.

Wendy Peebles had fits, proved by the psychiatrist to be completely hysterical. If there was no Wednesday night hop on in Tadchester, she came and had a fit in the middle of the surgery for a change. The rest of the Wednesday-nighters loved her performance. I must admit that, in my early days, she did worry me. It took me some time to realise that I was able to get her to come round quickly if I threatened her with a hypodermic needle or a bowl of cold water.

Mr Terence, the butcher's assistant, came regularly for stomach medicine and to talk about fly fishing. I had a feeling that it was damp river banks that gave him his indigestion, as it was quite clear he only took his medication at weekends.

Mrs Price, who worked in the supermarket, had anaemia. This was somehow related to the heavy floods of some years earlier. She used to love to describe the floods in such detail that I thought of saving up and buying her an ark. I daren't suggest that she had her womb taken away: it would have left her with one thing less – or perhaps one thing more – to talk about. She really would have liked a blood test each week as some kind of blanket insurance against anaemia, floods and hysterectomies. ('There can't be a drop of blood left in me, doctor.') As a sort of optional extra she would bring in her young son to show off his football bruises.

Jack Fingleton was a regular once-a-fortnight Wednesday-nighter. His wants were simple – some back tablets, a pound of cotton wool, and the largest bottle of liquid paraffin. He had been getting the cotton wool and oil before I came and he was such a regular that I didn't like to ask him what he used them for.

I got to know this group of patients so well that I began to remember them not by their names but by their conditions. On one embarrassing occasion at a cocktail party, I called George Ramsdale, my regular piles attender, 'Mr Bottom'.

The others were, variously, 'Mrs Varicose Ulcer', 'It's Me 'Art, You Know, Doctor', and 'Mrs It Keeps Dropping Down And I Can't Hold Me Water'.

At the time I was trying to adjust to this bizarre collection of patients and conditions, as if they weren't enough, I had two brushes with the Army. Retired Army officers, like private patients, I found difficult to get on with.

The first was Colonel Lotus. He came to see me in the surgery instead of consulting my senior partner, Steve Maxwell, who was his usual doctor. This was always a bad start. He came in, sat down and, in his clipped military manner, said, 'I'm afraid Maxwell's not up to it. I want you to look after me from now on.'

I should be able to have some trite and ready answer to squash retired military people, but I usually find that I am ill at ease with them. They bring out some hidden complex in me, and I am never able to deliver any prepared squelch. For a patient to say that Dr Maxwell was not up to it could only mean that there was something disagreeable about the patient himself.

I enquired about Colonel Lotus's trouble. He clipped out that he had had this damned neuritis for some years and that Maxwell had done nothing about it – what was I going to do?

I looked through his record card and saw the various investigations he had undergone. There was obviously nothing very seriously wrong, so I gave him a well-known brand of

84

vitamin tablets and told him to come back and see me in a fortnight's time.

When he returned in two weeks, in spite of his fierce look, he was almost pleasant – I didn't realise he had it in him.

'Damned good pills, those, doctor,' he said. 'Feel better than I've done for years. Wish I'd come to see you years ago. Let's have some more.'

I was pleased that he was going to be satisfied with vitamin tablets and gave him another prescription.

An hour later he rang up, irate.

'You've given me the wrong pills, doctor,' he bellowed. 'Damned inefficiency. Let me have some more of the ones you gave me last time. Did me the world of good.'

I consulted his card (I often have a horrible feeling that

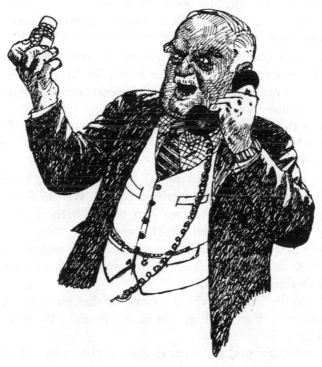

when I allow my mind to wander with a verbose patient, I will write down the wrong thing). I once wrote '3 The Elms' as the diagnosis part of a Health Certificate.

The other area in prescribing and writing certificates where I often lapsed was on the prescription form itself. In the top left-hand corner it says 'Mr/Mrs/Miss', two of which titles have to be struck out, depending on the sex and marital status of the patient concerned. In my speed of writing I often just took a wild slash at this group of prefixes, and my slashing was not always accurate. One day I was rung up by a mother who said that the elastic stockings I had prescribed for her baby's nappy rash didn't make sense, and the zinc and castor oil ointment I had given her for her varicose veins didn't help at all.

All it had on the Colonel's card was the vitamin tablets I was sure I had prescribed. I had to ring him back, and ask if he still had a tablet that he could let me see.

'Disgusting,' he said, under his breath. 'Damned records – I'll drop one in.'

At lunch time Gladys brought me a greyish-looking tablet that I was sure I had never seen in my life before. This is it, I thought – I must have prescribed the mental equivalent of '3 The Elms' in tablet form.

Even though this pill was apparently doing good, I didn't know what hidden harm it might be doing. I said to Gladys, 'We must find out what this is.'

We looked through his notes, without success, to see if it was something we had prescribed before. We checked it with every capsule and tablet we had in the surgery, and with every one of the coloured pill charts we kept.

I was in despair. I couldn't name this tablet, and the complex I have about treating retired colonels was very much to the fore. I didn't know what to do.

Eventually I rang Neville Jackson, the chemist, and explained my problem. 'Pop it round, old man,' he said. 'We'll soon find out what it is.'

I popped it round and went through all his stock – to no avail.

86

There didn't seem to be anything anywhere like it. We checked again, and still no identification. This really seemed like the end. The colonel was coming in to collect his pills in another half hour. We sat, and Neville said, 'Just a second – it couldn't possibly be ... you would never prescribe those ...' With my face getting redder, I said 'What?'

He went off to the veterinary counter and came back with a box of cats' worming tablets, opened it and showed me about fifty of the same tablets I was supposed to have prescribed. I hurried back to the surgery.

When the Colonel burst in, I was sitting with quiet dignity in my chair.

'Have you found out what those pills were? Disgusting – sheer inefficiency, bad book work, muddling things up. Never happened in the Army.'

'Sit down, Colonel,' I said, 'I've one or two questions to ask you.' He sat down, snorting.

'When you visited me last,' I said, 'were you alone?'

'What do you mean, alone?' he snorted. 'Of course I was.'

'No, no,' I said. 'Did you have any of your animals – the dogs, or cats – in the car?'

'Yes, yes,' he replied. 'I was taking the cat to the vet's – needed de-worming. Dashed good job he made of it, too.'

'I'm afraid, Colonel,' I said, 'the administrative mix-up has been on your part. The tablets that have done you so much good were the cat's worming tablets, and the tablets that have done the cat so much good were the ones I gave you!'

Colonel Lotus sat up sharply, as if he had been bayoneted in a tender spot. 'Ugh!' he exclaimed, then sat there silently, looking into space.

I left him in his trance for a few minutes, then enquired, 'Are you all right, Colonel?'

He replied with another 'Ugh', got up, and walked rather than stamped out of the surgery. I think for the first time in his whole life he simply had nothing he could say.

... General Branton did not attend the surgery, but was Army to the core, He fought his battles on his home ground.

To visit him was sheer hard work. The General, who had been famous for his exploits on the North West Frontier, campaigned just as vigorously against his bowels as he did against the Frontier tribesmen.

When I arrived he always had detailed communiqués of his actions of the last fourteen days. We then set out a working plan for the next fourteen days.

'What if I don't go tomorrow, and say I haven't been by Tuesday, and what happens if nothing really comes by Thursday?'

We waged an unremitting war against his bowels. It was important that we should never either win or lose completely, as he would have little else to live for. It was considered a reverse if we had to bring in the District Nurse to give an enema, whereas in the soft fruit season we sometimes had ten days of triumph.

I found, as time passed, that it had become less tedious. Like everything else, after a certain time you begin to get involved, start talking the same language. I began to get launched into his bowel manoeuvres just as intently as the General did, using suppositories and every conceivable laxative as my support troops.

Next door to the General lived Miss Wells, aged seventy-eight, who looked after her mother of 102. Her mother nagged her and chided her about not keeping the house clean, and not cooking as she used to. Although she was seventy-eight, Miss Wells behaved as if she were a young daughter and tried to improve her cooking and her scrubbing.

They lived very nearly at the top of Up the Hill. I used to see Miss Wells trudging with her shopping basket down the hill, across the bridge to the Pannier Market where she bought their weekly groceries and vegetables. Mother had always bought her stuff from the market, so poor Miss Wells had to follow suit.

She did confess to me one day in a moment of great weakness

that if the good Lord did take her mother away, perhaps she would at last have a little bit of life of her own.

Whereas General Branton's digestive tract represented the bottom end of the scale, the eating habits of the Tadchester patients (which are again quite unique) could probably be called the top end of the scale.

I had been called to *The Goat*, one of the larger pubs in Tadchester, to see the son of the landlord who was suffering from earache. I examined him, found that one of his ears was inflamed, and prescribed some antibiotics.

The landlord's wife asked, as I was there, whether I would mind having a look at the landlord himself, who had been complaining of indigestion.

The family had been in Tadchester for a few months only and I did not know the landlord very well. He was about twenty-nine but was already beginning to put on weight and would soon be able to make a matching pair with Bessie Oldthorpe.

I asked him about his symptoms, which seemed little more than some flatulence and a bit of epigastric discomfort.

'How much do you drink?' I asked.

'I really don't drink at all, doctor,' he replied, 'and if I do it's only light ale.'

This puzzled me: his symptoms sounded like an overdose of alcohol.

'On a market day,' he told me, 'I probably have about thirty short ales, but there are some days when I don't have more than about a dozen.'

He was obviously going to fit in well in Tadchester. For sheer peculiarity I would back the eating and drinking habits of Tadchesterians against those of any other town.

In my early days I treated two ladies for some peculiar disease for months without any effect, eventually calling in a specialist. I discovered they were eating a patent diet that they had read about in a national newspaper. It was completely devoid of Vitamin C and they were actually suffering from scurvy.

Mrs de Wyrebock's illness had shown me that raw sausage meat was a popular local delicacy and there were few Tadchester households which did not include a handful of seaweed with their morning bacon and egg. Eating too much was the general order of the day and I was plagued with overweight patients, none of whom, of course, ever ate a thing. One offender not only complained that I did nothing about reducing her weight, but loudly asserted that she vomited back every morsel of food she had taken for the last six months, and what was I going to do about it?

I tried every known slimming tablet and reducing diet on my gang of heavyweights but nothing happened. I asked Steve, 'Whatever do I do with all these fatties? Have you any favourite pill that works wonders?'

'I don't use pills,' said Steve. 'Just get them to write down every single thing they eat and drink each day for two weeks, then bring the list of their menus in to you.'

I followed Steve's instructions to the letter. My patients who never ate anything and were always putting on weight were instructed to make a complete diary of their food and drink intake and report back in a fortnight.

I weighed them all before they set out on this venture and again when they reported back with the mealtime records. It was amazing. There was an average weight loss of seven pounds per patient.

I was beginning to learn the art of general practice.

9

Formulae for Survival

I learned from my patients that only a few rare people have such a zest for life that they can cope unaided with all situations and seemingly survive them. Most people have to find some formula or philosophy of survival.

Often the formula was the discipline of a job. Just as often it was a hobby such as pigeon fancying, fishing or gardening. Life was the hobby: the daily grind of a job was endured merely to provide the means by which the hobby could be pursued. Other people were so weighed down with commitments that the commitments themselves were a formula. Ties of elderly sick relatives or young children decided for them how they were going to spend most of their lives – they had no option.

It was how people behaved when released from their commitments that amazed me. Far from entering a much wider and fuller life, more often they fell to pieces. The Harris family were typical of this group.

Granny Harris was the bane of her family's life. She had had a stroke and could not communicate properly, was intermittently incontinent, and had to be fed and washed. It was an unrewarding chore the family had shared strictly between them for ten years. They had promised her at some stage before her stroke that if she was ever ill they would never put her into hospital. They stuck to their word.

Eventually winter bronchitis took her off. She had led a cabbage-like uncommunicative existence for so long I felt I could not give her antibiotics to see this particular phase through. She died peacefully in her sleep, to what must, I felt, have been a great joy to her family.

The Harris's were one of the large local Tadchester families, so there was a splendid funeral. Although there were some outward signs of grief, it must have been a tremendous relief to all of them. They were close-knit and had shared, uncomplainingly, the task of nursing Granny between four of the households, each taking a three-month stint. Other members of the family saw to it that they were adequately relieved to go out and join in normal communal life as far as they possibly could. They were a great example of people looking after their own.

Within three months of Granny dying the family had more or less split up. They did not bother with each other any more; there were quarrels, gossip, and some sections of the family were not on speaking terms with others. I found it difficult to believe that Granny Harris, this immobile invalid, must have been the cornerstone of the family structure. Once she had gone the whole building had tumbled down.

Even more surprising was Charlie Leggo. He was in his seventies when I came to the practice and had been nursing his elderly parents at home for some years. His mother was in her very late eighties and his father ninety-two.

He washed them, powdered them, fed and clothed them. They were still just mobile when I first came to Tadchester but gradually deteriorated and were both confined to bed.

I never enquired too closely into how their toilet was managed, but they were both impeccably looked after, without a blemish on them. Charlie, who was an odd-fish bachelor, never grumbled about how much he had to do for them. He had spent most of his life with his parents. They had had a family butcher's shop in the town. Apart from a brief interlude in the Army in the First World War, Charlie had worked in, and later managed, the shop. He finally shut it when he was about sixty-three, only because the demands of his parents took up all his time.

His father, the weaker of the two ancients, eventually died.

Charlie took it in his stride because his main love was his mother, and he was now able to devote all his time to her.

There was never a better nurse. He attended to her every whim, washed her, powdered her, rubbed her hands when they were cold, and would buy any tempting morsel of food that she might fancy, irrespective of cost.

Although Charlie wandered about all day in a brown overall and looked as poor as a church mouse, it was rumoured that he had tens of thousands of pounds in a case under his bed. I could quite believe this as he never appeared to spend anything on himself and it wouldn't have surprised me if he had pinched his brown overalls when he was discharged from the Army in 1919.

Six months later, in spite of Charlie's ministrations, his mother died. I wondered how he would adjust to living on his own.

He spent the first few months weeping, not leaving the house, castigating himself – and me – for not having taken greater care of his parents. Couldn't I have given her some different medicine? Was the medicine I had given them the right medicine? I, meanwhile, tried to urge him to get out and actually accused him of going nowhere and suggested I would have to get a psychiatrist in to see him.

'I do go out,' said Charlie. 'I go to all the funerals of the regular customers we used to have at the shop.'

Slowly Charlie began to take some interest in life. By 'interest in life' I mean 'interest in himself'. Now, relieved of his domestic duties, he had little to do other than prowl around his body looking for untreatable or incurable illnesses.

The only time he was away from his parents, during the First World War, he received a leg injury on the Somme which left him with a varicose ulcer that had withstood every medical treatment for several decades. His ulcer was really his pride and joy. Once, trying out some new technique, I did almost cure it.

93

From then on Charlie kept it tightly bandaged and wouldn't let me look at it.

One of his explorations brought to light a previously un-discovered cyst on his posterior, approximately the size of a garden pea. It was a nuisance, and would have to be removed. This was out of my province and would require his going to the outpatients' department at the hospital, where Henry Johnson would attend to it.

To my surprise Charlie accepted the idea of going to hospital with enthusiasm; he was living the life of a recluse now and rarely left the house. He was a martinet in his own home and vented most of his spleen on his home help who always did more than her duty, hoping that one day she might be remembered in his will.

I wondered how Charlie would get on at the hospital. He had always been so used to getting his own way. He had no great experience of hospital staff to help him dominate them but, to his eternal credit, he triumphed. The fierce theatre sister was handled more firmly than she had ever been in her life before, and Charlie went down in history as the only man to mount the hospital theatre table without first removing his boots.

When he was actually installed on the table, plus boots, it was with great difficulty that he was persuaded to lift his shirt so that the offending lesion could be admired.

As the operation was under local anaesthetic, Charlie was able to talk all the way through, dropping titbits of medical information, and refusing to come back and have his stitches out in seven days as he knew they should stay in for nine. Henry said afterwards he nearly put a stitch in his tongue.

When they were putting on his dressing, Charlie finally won the day. With a triumphant look in his eye he said, 'I shall need some physiotherapy for this.' How, why and from whatever angle I was never to know: three days after the operation he suddenly packed up and went south to live with a niece no one had heard of, and he never appeared again.

In complete contrast to the Harris's and Charlie Leggo,

Mrs Saunders was one of the happy few who seemed to survive without any particular formula. She was the respected, gentle wife of one of the Methodist lay preachers who lived Up the Hill. In addition to looking after her aged mother-in-law for ten years, she kept a spotless house and took meals in to the poverty-stricken lady who lived next door. The poverty-stricken lady next door, Miss Rudd, accepted any charity that was going (including the Christmas dinner at a local hotel that I arranged one year). She surprised us all when she died by leaving her dirty, untidy house almost crammed to the roof with share certificates, £1 notes, and Savings Certificates, to a total value of £37,000. This was not including the value of the house she lived in, which was her own.

Miss Rudd had died intestate, and a tentative enquiry was put out for any possible living beneficiaries.

Far from having no family, she appeared to have a vast one: relatives started to appear from all over England, to put a claim in for dear Auntie Gertie's fortune.

There were two devoted nephews and one niece actually living in Tadchester. They had apparently not managed to bring themselves to visit her for ten or fifteen years, but underneath really loved her dearly, and each one of the Tadchester three were quite sure that it was them in particular who Auntie would have loved to leave her money to.

I was happy that it was the solicitors who would have to sort this lot out.

Eventually Mrs Saunders' mother-in-law died and Mrs Saunders was left free to devote more of her time to the running and organising of the church that her husband was associated with. She had always somehow kept herself intact and not bowed down by her commitments. She had very rarely attended the surgery, so when she did come to see me one day, complaining of stomach pain, I knew there must be something really upsetting her.

I always took extra notice of patients who, like Mrs Saunders, only rarely appeared at the surgery. If they had made a special

95

effort to come, it must have been for a good reason. Their medical record cards gave a great deal of information.

One man whose record card showed me he had not seen a doctor for twelve years came in for a bottle of medicine for his irritating cough. 'No need to examine me, doctor,' he said.

I did examine him, heard a few suspicious squeaks, and sent him for an X-ray of his chest. He had a cancer of the lung. Within six weeks of his seeing me, his lung had been removed.

It was the same situation with Mrs Saunders. She had obviously been having womb trouble for some time and, on my examination, I found that she had some internal growth.

I made an urgent appointment for her to be seen by the specialist. He admitted her to hospital within a week and carried out a major operation. In his letter to me afterwards he explained that, although he had removed most of the growth, the patient had really come to him too late, and there were signs that the growth was already beginning to spread.

Mrs Saunders, as expected, made a good recovery from her operation and for six months was out and about, brighter than ever.

Then came signs that her disease was beginning to catch up with her. She complained of increasing pain in her right leg – obviously the growth must have infiltrated the sciatic nerve of the affected side. She was requiring increasing quantities of drugs to relieve her pain, she wasn't eating, she was losing weight. Her pain was slowly killing her.

I hoped that we might be able to make her last weeks (or months) more comfortable and asked the consultant anaesthetist from Winchcombe Hospital if he would come over and see her. I felt that if he could kill the nerves in her leg (this could sometimes be done by injecting alcohol into it) it would make life more bearable for her, although it would not halt the progress of her disease.

The consultant anaesthetist came over and skilfully injected her leg. Twenty-four hours later, Mrs Saunders was completely pain-free, and eating properly again. Within two weeks, she was up and about, busying herself with town and church matters.

This was a marvellous response to treatment. I wondered how long it would be before her disease finally caught up with her.

Once she was free of pain, Mrs Saunders stopped attending me. There was no point in my reminding her that she had a very unpleasant medical condition.

Months and years slipped by and the details of her particular case became submerged in the mass of other problems I had to deal with.

Seven years later I was called to her house again. She had fallen down the stairs and broken her hip. She went into hospital, had her hip pinned, was home and walking again after two weeks, and never looked back.

The surgeon who pinned her hip said there were still signs of the growth but for some reason (I have no explanation for it) it hadn't advanced. Apart from some numbness in her leg where the nerves had been killed, she had no complaints.

I am sure that if her pain had not been relieved she would have died. I became aware that people do die of pain; that people in bad accidents have a much better chance of surviving if their pain is relieved. I also came to realise that if I predicted too closely the course a certain disease would take, I would be proved wrong as often as I was proved right.

Mrs Saunders' story was one of the happy rewards that I occasionally came across in general practice. Unfortunately, too often, there were events of great sadness.

Silas Lister was a recluse who lived in a flat over some garages near the quay on the Down the Hill side of the river. He kept himself to himself, rarely communicated with anyone, was reputed to have money but lived in a miserly fashion. He refused to accept things like electricity and gas, and would be found bundled in several layers of dirty old coats picking up driftwood from the side of the river when the tide was out. At night, through his curtainless windows, his flickering candle could be seen moving as he passed from room to room.

The Social Services made several offers to help him but he refused, was belligerent to anybody who approached him, and kept himself behind the locked door of his flat.

He did not appear for days sometimes, and the only evidence that there was still life in the flat was that the pint of milk delivered each day at some time disappeared inside. He had behaved in this way for as long as anyone could remember, and was of indeterminate age.

One day the milkman reported that no bottles had been taken in for three days: he could not get any reply when he knocked on the door, and felt that either Silas had gone away or was ill in his flat.

I went down but couldn't get any reply either, and there was no way of looking into the rooms as they were one storey up.

I called the police, who broke into the flat for me, and we were met by a scene of absolute carnage.

In one corner of a bare, untidy room lay the shrivelled and obviously dead body of Silas, but it looked as if there had been some terrible and bloody struggle. Blood literally covered the floor of virtually every room of the flat, with Silas's bare feet occasionally showing their imprint on the dark stains on the floorboards.

On closer examination there seemed to be no evidence of a struggle after all and, what was stranger still, in my brief examination of Silas I could find no evidence of where he had been bleeding from. He was thin – almost emaciated – and obviously undernourished, with spindly legs and huge varicose veins running down both ankles.

It was a complete mystery.

I went to the post mortem and the mystery was solved.

The pathologist showed me the cause of Silas's downfall. There was a small hole in one varicose vein on one of Silas's ankles. He must have caught his ankle while wandering about in the dark, or semi-dark, of his flat, and pottered about, slowly letting his life blood drain away. You would have thought that he would have been conscious that the floor was wet and sticky, but we were never quite sure how much Silas was conscious of anything, and in some strange way this is probably the way Silas would have chosen to go – a slow ebbing out of his life force, painlessly, and followed by a long and lasting sleep.

In any other circumstance, one small dressing or a finger pressed on this tiny wound would have stopped the bleeding.

IO

Down the Mine

It became my lot to take over the surgeries at Thudrock Colliery.

I liked coal miners and looked forward to my excursions to the primitive surgery that we had there.

Coal mining was in my blood. My grandfather had been a collier, my father had been a coal mining engineer, until his untimely death, and at the end of the war I had had two years down a mine as a Bevin Boy.

One·of the factors that made me choose the Winchcombe area was that it was one of the very few parts of Britain which had the benefits of the south of England and its better weather, the sea coast, and a coal mine not too far away.

The Thudrock miners loved having a doctor who was a qualified collier, who could talk the same language and knew all about the perils of the coal face and underground roadways. The few I was unpopular with were the lead swingers who failed to put it across me because I knew it all – even a bit more than some of them.

I was taken on trips underground, up to the coal face, and felt a strange nostalgia for the time when my daily task was with a pick and shovel in a 3 foot 6 inch seam.

* * *

As a medical student, I had volunteered to go down the mines. In December 1944, six of us were sitting in the Biology Lab. in Epsom College. We were a sub-section of the Medical Six who had been sitting the first M.B. and the Conjoint Board Premedical Examination. These were our last few days as schoolboys. The war was pressing on to its conclusion; we were too young and isolated to appreciate its horrors, and indulged in schoolboy fugues of heroism and daring acts. None of us wanted to go straight away to Medical School. We had opted as one man for the Fleet Air Arm where, with pride, we'd learnt that the average life of a pilot in the air was thirty-six hours. What would they think at the Youth Club when we came in in our uniforms?

I discussed the situation with my mother, who always kept me on a loose rein. She thought some experience before Medical School would be valuable, that the Fleet Air Arm certainly sounded glamorous, but the way things were going the war would soon be over, and that the chances of reaching air crew would be virtually nil: I would be wasting my time for a few years doing some mundane job. If I really wanted to do something valuable which would widen my experience and make a contribution to society, why not go down the mines for a year? The Bevin Scheme was under way at the time and men were being conscripted for the mines as they were the Armed Forces.

I have a streak in me, that has persisted, of doing the out-of-the-ordinary. The mines caught my imagination. So I went to the Labour Exchange and asked if I could go down the pit for a year. They said they would be delighted to have me – as a medical student I could come out when I liked – and so I signed on there and then. My mother's wisdom prevailed: my five friends went into the Fleet Air Arm, spent five months making paths across airfields with clinker and coke, and were then given an early discharge. Thus, on 1st February 1945, I set out for Doncaster with a bright Ministry of Labour label on my case.

Proudly flashing the label as if it were a D.S.C. or at least a Captain's pips, I reached Askern Main Colliery, one of the main initial training establishments for Bevin Boys in the Yorkshire coalfields.

I was at Askern for a month, part of a very mixed bunch. With my Boy Scout's enthusiasm, I could not understand why my colleagues were not delighted to be able to go down pits and dig out coal. Most of them were either from industry where, with the reduction in arms production, they had become redundant and had been conscripted for the mines, or were air crew, many of whom had been training in Canada where there was a reduction in personnel with the war drawing to a close. When I look back and think of the adjustment that these Officer Cadets had to make, one minute being feted in Canada in smart uniforms and with reasonable pay, then almost overnight being transformed into coal miners, I realise it must have been almost too much to bear.

There were one or two straight conscripts who were neither redundant factory workers nor ex-Air Force. These included a concert pianist and one poor lad who had never strayed from his father's estates, where he had a private tutor, his only glimpse of the public being when he was supervising hop-picking on the family estate. In one of our many political discussions – and this was at the time of the Socialist revolutions – poor 'Lord Tom' as he was called, in a very hostile environment put forward the suggestion that the only possible government was that of genuine aristocracy. On reflection, after thirty years, I think he was probably right.

In addition to the change of circumstances, for most of my fellow Bevin Boys there was a marked reduction in the amount of money they had. Many had been making very good money working long hours as bench hands in Midlands factories.

We were good company. There were various dances and social engagements, and one of the local farmers asked a group of us round for ham and eggs in quantities that I had not seen since before the war.

We had our delightful eccentrics, two brothers who were the

sons of, and bore the name of, a famous cough-medicine manufacturer. They had a row with their father, and volunteered for the mines that day. They distinguished themselves when being posted to their pit near Nottingham by living at the most fashionable hotel in the town and crossing the lounge in the evening in their pit boots and helmets on their way to their rooms for a wash.

We were housed at Askern in the proverbial Army Nissen hut, with stoves, bunk beds and lockers. We ate at the pit canteen for lunch but came back to the hostel for our evening meal. Our day was split up between lectures, physical training and visits down the pit. The lectures were very simple, about life underground, and I still have the books that I won for being top in the examination. Physical training was the routine stuff with a regular ex-Guards sergeant.

Visits underground were quite different. This was a new experience for all of us. Half of the colliery was in production and the other half was used for the training of Bevin Boys. I never liked, and know of nobody who does like, going down in a pit cage. You hurtle down into the darkness to the accompaniment of the hissing of compressed air pipes and, usually, dripping water. With the slowing down of the cage at the bottom you feel you are shooting back up to the top again.

Only once had I been in a pit cage when anything unusual happened. On this occasion there was some technical fault. We had neared the bottom and then were lifted back up half-way, a quarter of a mile from daylight and quarter of a mile from the bottom. Tension mounted steadily. We were hopeless, helpless, and did not know what was going on. I could feel the tension rising. One cannot contemplate shinning up a quarter of a mile of rope, neither sliding down one. Happily, after ten minutes, we went down and were got off on to safe ground.

The training shaft at Askern Colliery had an added refinement in that there was a two-tier cage, of which only the top tier was used. The reason for this was apparent on our first trip. We huddled together as the cage sped down, thinking we were

103

almost certainly plunging to our deaths. The end of the journey finished in a loud splash which confirmed our worst fears. What in fact was happening was that the sump (which is the space below where the cage stops to unload in the pit bottom) was full of water into which the bottom tier of the cage used to splash to unload the top tier. It was all too much for our pianist who was claustrophobic and quite hysterical. He made two or three more attempts to go down the pit, but was eventually discharged as being unfit to serve underground.

We climbed along tunnels, through coal faces, spent half a day working in a place called Garsides, which was extremely hot. After four weeks, in which we had just got to know each other, we were split up and posted to various collieries in the South Yorkshire field. A few of us managed to stick together and were posted to Dinnington Main Colliery, near Sheffield. We had been living in hostels till now, and were transferred to another hostel (Nissen huts, bunk beds again) but were expected to find accommodation in Dinnington Village once we had settled in.

During our first month at Dinnington we were put through a hardening-up process, which meant that at six o'clock every morning we had to report at the pit top and unload a twenty-ton railway wagon full of stones or clinker. This was our day's work. Here we acquired our blisters and developed our shovelling muscles. As the old miner in charge of us said, 'If you shovel at an elephant's feet, it will fall over.'

One of the few things that has remained with me from my mining days is skill with a shovel. You aim always for a flat surface, and you start shovelling at the bottom.

I managed to find lodgings in Dinnington with a collier and his wife with whom I stayed happily for two years. We still keep in touch – Auntie and Ike Bradley, who gave me full board, lodging, laundry, love and care for twenty-five shillings (£1.25p) a week.

Toughened up, I was ready to work underground. I hated my first job down below. It was working in the pit bottom, assisting in putting tubs on and off the cage. It was cold, noisy and relentless. There seemed to be streams of tubs loaded with coal coming at you all the time. You stopped a tub by pushing what was known as a 'locker' between the spokes of the running wheel, which acted as an instant brake. You had to be careful not to put your hand in or under the wheel, and if you missed with your locker a stream of tubs could come pouring down, smashing the cage and halting the drawing of coal. As far as I remember the drawing rate was sixty times an hour: one only had a few seconds to unload a tub, push the empty tubs off the cage with the full tubs, shut the gates and leap back. There were horrific tales told of men catching their sleeves in the up-going cage, and I hated it.

There are two shafts in a coal mine: one the down shaft in which the air is drawn into the mine, and the other the up shaft where the stale, but now warm, air is drawn out. I was at the bottom of the down shaft. In mid-winter it was very cold.

I had come to be a coal miner and would settle for nothing less than a pick and shovel. I was only going to be down a year, and I wanted to do the whole lot. Colliers were the fighter pilots of the industry. They were the real men who had a confident swagger, knowing that whatever anybody else did, they were the men that mattered and the rest were just supporting troops. When eventually I was a collier myself, I likened the experience very much to that of the small amount of rock climbing that I had done; there is the same physical effort, some hazard, and the sense of achievement and accomplishment at the end of the day.

After four weeks on the pit bottom I was moved to a job further in the pit which was reckoned to be one of the softest jobs going. In a little airless side passage we had a compressed-air prop-straightening machine. Nearly all the pit props and roof supports – bars – were iron. The bent and twisted ones were brought off the coal faces to be straightened in this machine.

I was Ben Burgess's assistant. He was an old collier, past retiring age, a great character, who was delighted to have a medical student as his sidekick. The job was tedious to the extreme. It was so hot and airless that it was very difficult to keep awake: the job had no incentive. Sometimes we would run out of props and bars and would sit, fighting to keep awake. The worst sin you can commit underground is to fall asleep. It is a bit like falling asleep in the snow – you may never wake up.

We had visits from the deputies (foremen) and the overman (foreman in charge of underground shift) who would pass the time of day with us. The few remaining pit ponies – under-worked, overfed, savage beasts – used to come with their terrified drivers to carry our props away in small trucks. The pit ponies that I saw didn't need anybody to feel sorry for them. They did little work, were extremely well fed and looked after, were extremely difficult to control, and were, proverbially, as strong as a horse.

My friend Albert, who is now a successful Birmingham jeweller, came flying past one day, hanging on to the bit of his aggressive pony, not being able to stop him for a further half mile, with always the danger that the pony would pull the tub off the rails and bring down the roof of the narrow underground passages – 'supply gates' – through which they travelled. They were only about five feet in height – tall enough for the pony but not the driver.

My days with Ben seemed to go on for ever. If you have been half asleep in a boring lecture you know the agony of being nine hours a day in this situation. Ben warned me of the perils of the coal face. I had a safe job with him, but I wanted the coal face – the complete experience. So, after only two months underground, I was offered the job of coal face borer.

A coal face borer was by far the worst job – at least for me – on the coal face. It hadn't the sheer strain and exhaustion of actually getting coal, but the frustrations and the difficult positions one had to get into more than made up for this.

In 1945, face drills were driven by compressed air and there was a compressed-air pipe the whole length of the face. This was covered with lumps of loose coal, coal dust, and had coupling valves every fifteen to twenty yards. The face borer had first to blow out any dust from the pipes without getting his head blown off, then with a six-foot drill and thirty yards of rubber tubing, had to scramble up and down the coal face as the colliers requested holes for blowing their coal. He had to find the valves hidden in the dust, make sure his machine did not jam, make sure that he had sharp bits for his drill – and all this while carrying a hand lamp.

It was the nearest to Dante's inferno that I have been. There was the noise of falling coal, dust, shouts and screams of the colliers who wanted 'the bloody borer', and acrid smoke following the face as shots were fired further along it. If the shot had not been placed in deeply enough (a flanker) the whole face became thick with blinding smoke.

On some faces the conveyor belt was put right up to the coal face and the collier had to dig a hole in for himself to get working. The poor borer had to travel up and down this three-hundred-yard length, hopping in and out of the waste behind the coal face that might come down at any minute, clamber over the conveyor belt with huge lumps of coal trying to knock him off all the time, and perch sometimes across the belt with coal whizzing between his legs as he fought to drill a six-foot hole into the coal. His other duties were to put props, clay for shot firing, and wooden nogs (which were used to stop props slipping) on the end of the face belts so the colliers could pull supplies off for themselves as the material passed them. It was an absolute nightmare. You were nobody's friend.

On my first day as a borer I was sent to Five's Face where the coal was thicker than anywhere else in the pit, being about five feet from roof to floor, and getting about was rather easier. Half way through my first shift I saw everyone down tools and get off the face very quickly. I thought 'Ah! snap (lunch) time,' and wandered slowly off the face, surprised at the noise of the creaking and grinding of the roof. I was even more surprised when the coal face behind me started to burst, shooting lumps of coal right across the belt. Only when I got off the face and somebody grabbed me, not too politely, did I realise there was what was known as a dreaded 'top weight' on: a major rock subsidence which can squash a coal face flat – in spite of props, timbers and bars – in a matter of minutes. This was the only top weight I experienced in more than two years underground, and I was too naive to know its implications.

I was a coal face borer for three months, itching to have a go with pick and shovel. I would be paid more, and there was always something degrading about being a borer; how much you were at people's beck and call, how the whole face could be at a standstill if you did not get your pipes blown out.

At last the great day came.

'No borers needed on Fives. You can have a go at a stint, Bob lad,' said the Deputy. Pleased as Punch, I swaggered off with my pick and heart-shaped shovel. I was going to be a collier at last.

My first stint was on Three's face, which had a certain notoriety. It had bad roof faults which made timbering and propping difficult and had slips where the coal cut narrowed out, and rock and coal had to be taken together. It was also the furthest face out – one had to walk one and a half miles uphill along a narrow low supply road to the face – it was also the hottest.

We used to walk to the face in our pit clothes. Trousers, jacket and, for some reason, waistcoat were always fashionable underground. But working gear comprised solely a pair of short cotton pants, heavy pit safety boots with metal toecaps, and fibre pit helmets. Although head lamps with the battery attached to the waist were becoming the fashion, we had only heavy, electric hand lamps, like miniature lighthouses. One man in six also carried an oil lamp for gas testing.

Working at the coal face on a stint was by far the hardest work I have ever experienced. We arrived at the coal face at six o'clock and I eventually cleared my stint with the help of a collier in the next stint by two o'clock. There was no stopping for lunchtime breaks – just an occasional swig at the water bottle and a terrible race of flashing shovels, flying coal, back-breaking putting up of metal bars with metal props which, if not put in properly, could fly out like catapults and maim you.

I was completely exhausted after my first shift. My friend, Albert, helped me on to the Paddy train and up in the lift cage. 'Stupid bugger,' he said. And this became my daily task. For sheer physical graft and endeavour I have never known its equal. It was hot, noisy, dusty, with smoke coming from shots being fired.

The work was always just a bit more than I could manage and Bill Whitely, in the next stint, very often had to help me out. It can't have pleased him because each stint was enough for any one man. At its easiest you got twelve tons of coal to shovel, push and lever on to the conveyor belt, but threequarters of your shift could be spent getting your coal down and into workable-sized lumps. Occasionally I would arrive and things were just as they should be – the coal had blown through to the back; this meant that all the loose coal (gumming) had been cleared out before the shot had fired. Some of my Bevin Boy friends on the previous shift knew my stint number and looked after me as best they could.

I was on a stint continually from June 1945 till December 1946. It was completely exhausting work, but had a particular satisfaction that I have never met elsewhere. Once you were finished, you were finished: the next day brought a fresh battle but each day brought a fresh achievement, and you left the battlefield and went to a world outside.

Some time in 1945 I had a letter from the Ministry of Labour giving me a number, inferring that I would be doing a full stint of National Service. I made no protest about our original agreement. It seemed only fair. Anticipating a discharge towards the end of 1947, I applied for admission to a teaching hospital in London.

I went down to London for an interview – the only professional collier they had considered. To my surprise, not long after I got back, I received a letter from the Dean saying that they were creating a number of places for ex-service men in January 1947; they had applied to the Ministry of Labour for my release, but had been turned down.

At the last Mineworkers' Union meeting I had been to, and knowing that I was applying for a hospital, the officials said, 'Don't you worry, Bob lad. As soon as they offer you a place in the hospital, we'll see you get your release.' I took my Dean's letter to the N.U.M. and on the 28th December 1946 I received a letter from the Ministry of Labour saying that I could go.

I did my last shift, and forty-eight hours later had started at the hospital as a medical student. But this was not to be the end of mining for me. It was in my blood.

In the long vacation of the summer of 1947, the Coal Board fixed me up with a pit in Nottingham – Rufford Colliery, near Mansfield. I stayed in a theatrical boarding house, missing Caroll Levis's Discoveries by one week. I was on the haulage for a week to acclimatise myself to underground conditions and then spent the next six weeks working on the coal face. I worked with a collier in the corner of the face where the coal was some distance from the belt and had to be thrown in two moves – the collier to me, and then me to the belt. I soon rediscovered a few muscles that I had forgotten, and collected a fine set of blisters.

After six weeks I came back fit and strong for the beginning of the rugby season. It was the most rigorous training I had ever done.

In 1949 I again went back to the pits in the long summer vacation, this time to Bolsover Colliery in Derbyshire.

At Bolsover I had a week in an eighteen-inch seam where they were heading out a new face. The face was so low that you either shovelled on your stomach or came off from the face and returned on your back. There was no room for your pelvis between the roof and the floor.

A week of this was plenty for me, but some men, particularly in the Durham coalfields, spent their lives working in these conditions.

I had thought at one time of doing industrial medicine, but found that I would have to spend most of my time checking first-aid boxes in pit canteens and doing routine medical inspections. General practice was the thing I was destined for.

One morning in my surgery at Thudrock a miner came in and asked if he could sign on as a temporary resident. There was something slightly familiar about his face, but his cap was pulled well down over his eyes. He didn't begin to fill in the temporary resident's form, but just stood, staring at the table.

'How can I help you?' I asked.

He pulled up his right trouser leg, and there was a round blue scar, plumb in the middle of his calf.

'Is it hurting?' I asked.

'No,' grunted the collier. 'I just wondered if I should sue the man who did it.'

He looked up, grinning. It was Albert Catts, one of the deputies at Dinnington Colliery, where I had spent my two years. I had given him that scar.

One day on the coal face, swinging away with my lightweight pick, I had not heard Albert come up behind me and had swung my pick straight into his leg. His language had finally completed my education.

It was marvellous to see him again, and we had a very beery evening at the Miners' Institute – a place I found difficult to get away from without drinking my weight in beer.

I was to be the medical officer at Thudrock Colliery for many years, and made many friends there. The good times I had with the colliers were balanced with the accidents that I had to deal with, but down the pit – that's life.

11

The Nightmare

I was at Winchcombe on my half day off, doing some shopping, when the fire took place.

I arrived back in Tadchester to find the town stunned, and a pall of smoke still hanging over the school. People were walking about, stern faced, not talking, not smiling.

Three ten-year-olds at the large secondary school had broken into the senior laboratory during the lunch hour to make some stink bombs – or so their friends said. Whatever they had done, they had started some conflagration which had trapped them, and all three had been burnt to death.

It was just frightful, and nobody could bear to think about it. All three families were patients of Steve Maxwell's so, thank God, I wasn't the one to have to go round and do the comforting.

I could think of no one better than Steve, with his kindly presence and gentle ways, to be with them and help them cope with this awful situation.

These were the times when Steve was at his best. There was a saintliness about him. He was painstaking, unselfish in what he did. A bachelor, his life was medicine and his patients were his children.

I slept badly that night, thinking of this terrible tragedy, and worrying about how the families would have to cope and live with it.

There was a very small surgery the next morning. For once people were not thinking much about themselves – they were more concerned with the tragedy that had fallen on the community.

I was surprised to get a call from the police midway through the morning, asking me if I would go down to the mortuary. They thought they would need me there, they said.

I was led into the mortuary by a red-eyed constable, who was nervous, apprehensive, and ill at ease.

'The mothers have to identify the bodies,' he said. 'We thought that they ought to have a doctor with them.'

Normally the police would have sufficed, but it was just all too much for this particular constable. Oh God, I thought. Am I going to be able to bear all this?

I looked through the glass into the waiting room and could see the three mothers waiting patiently to undergo this ghastly ordeal. Two of them I knew slightly, the other I hadn't seen before. All three sat with their heads bowed, not talking; perhaps unaware of, or not having come to terms with, this horrific situation.

'Would you like to go in on your own for a bit first?' said the constable.

He opened the door, and then shut it behind me. He certainly didn't want to go in there again.

In the room were four trestle tables, over three of which were stretched white sheets, silhouetting the small bodies that they covered. I lifted each sheet and looked at the charred remains of what were, yesterday, happy, playing children. It was awful. The tears were running down my cheeks. How was I going to face this?

I dried my eyes, composed myself, went back to the door and said, 'Perhaps the first mother would like to come in.'

Fortunately there had been some reasonable degree of identification from the clothes, and I was not, I hoped, going to have to expose these mothers to the sight of three destroyed children.

The first woman came in. She was the one I didn't know. It

was ghastly. I just couldn't relate to being there. She was ashen, trembling and nervous, clasping her hands tightly round the strap of her handbag.

I shut the door behind her. I said, 'My dear, there's only you and me here. There is no need for you to see your child if you don't want to. I am quite prepared to vouch that you have seen her.'

'No,' said the woman. 'I must see my little Emma. It would have been her eleventh birthday tomorrow.' As she said this the tears started to course down her face.

I walked over to the table on which we thought were the remains of her daughter, and lifted back the sheet.

'Oh God! No!' she cried.

I caught her just before she fell to the floor.

I covered the remains of her child with a sheet. I put my arms round her, and she clasped me, then after a few minutes, composed herself.

She stood up, wiped her eyes, said, 'Thank you, doctor,' and let herself out of the room.

I just had to sit down. I called the policeman and said, 'Have you a cigarette?' He didn't come through the door but handed me a packet, and I smoked a cigarette before I could face the ordeal of the second mother.

Both the other two mothers in turn, as they came through the door, clung to me – I knew them slightly. Both were frightened to look at these terrible white mounds that confronted them. In each case I again said, as I had with the first, that I would swear that they had identified their child. There was no need for them to look if they didn't want to. But both insisted they should have a last look at what once had been their happy child. I had to support both of them in turn with my arm.

It seemed to go on for ever.

The last mother, having had to wait for the first two to finish their inspection, collapsed completely and we had to call an ambulance to take her home.

For some reason it was the mothers who had come to do this

worst of all jobs, not the fathers. Perhaps children are closer to their mothers, or mothers closer to their children. I knew two of the fathers and they were fine men, neither of whom would shirk their responsibilities.

God, how do people stand these situations? How could I advise them what to do in this sort of catastrophe? I would not have been able to cope if it had been a child of mine. What right had I to advise and tell them what to do, or try and give them some trite word of comfort?

Perhaps the situation makes the man. I don't know. I only hoped that I would never ever have to be tested in circumstances like these myself.

The morning had been a nightmare. I somehow managed, tight lipped, to get myself out of the building after I had seen the mothers away. I got into my car in a daze and drove a couple of miles out of the town.

I parked in a lay-by, put my head on my knees, and wept.

12

Miracles and Malingerers

In my early days in practice I became very much aware of how much people's personalities affected both their chance of recovery and speed of recovery. Patients who were determined to die, most often did. I had read of primitive tribesmen turning their faces to the wall and dying. I hadn't believed before that it could happen in what we call our civilised society, but it undoubtedly did.

I had Tadchester patients who made up their minds to die and then died, for no other reason than that they did not want to live.

I saw some miracles for which I had no explanation. Joyce Taylor, the wife of Jack Taylor, one of the local outfitters, developed an abdominal pain and a lump in her stomach. Henry opened her up and found she was riddled with cancer. It was quite inoperable. He stitched her up again, not having interfered at all, and after a stormy passage she got over her operation.

She was an intelligent woman who demanded to know the score. Had she got a cancer? Was it operable, and how long had she to live? She had plans to make.

When people asked me whether they were going to die I nearly always said no: this was the answer they were looking for. I found by experience that if you told patients that they had not long to live or that they had some incurable disease, this shortened the time they would have had with us. There were some people like Joyce Taylor who defied all the odds.

She planned out her six months and carried on quite normally. The six months spread into seven, then to eight, then it was a year since her operation. Henry used to see her from time to time and found the lump in her stomach was gradually disappearing. For no accountable reason, Joyce Taylor was still going on quite happily sixteen years after she had been told she had six months to live.

Morry Loudson was a rough diamond who kept a scrap yard down at the back of the railway station. Although he ostensibly made his money from collecting old metal, he was into every fiddle that was going. I am sure a few stolen cars went his way, as did a few rustled cattle and any deer that were unwise enough to stray within ten miles of Tadchester.

He came to the surgery to see Jack Hart with swollen legs and a swelling of the lower abdomen. He was investigated at the hospital and eventually had an exploratory operation, when it was found that he had a rare tumour of the inner muscles of the back. This type of cancer was inoperable, would not respond to drugs, and was insensitive to X-rays. He, again, was told the full score. He sold his scrap yard and decided that he would end his days in the happy oblivion of alcohol.

He became grossly swollen from the waist down and could hardly walk. It was difficult to say if it were just his swollen legs that were limiting his walking as he always had a shipload of booze on board. One day he was found drunk and unconscious at the side of the road and had to be brought into hospital, have his head stitched, and be kept under observation for a few days.

He was given some drugs to get rid of the excess fluid in his legs, was deprived of alcohol for a week and, with a reduction of his swelling, he began to look more like a human being. He cheerfully discharged himself after seven days and then, like Mrs Taylor, suddenly began to get better. After two years, with no money left from the sale of his scrap yard, he took on a job as a brickie's mate with one of the local builders and, as far as

I know, never looked back – except to make absolutely sure that the pub doors were firmly shut.

'Blessed are the meek for they shall inherit the earth' was certainly sometimes true about patients. If a patient in the hospital was a pleasant, likeable person who got on well with the nursing staff and caused as little trouble as possible, then the nursing staff were all over him and would go much more out of their way to help him than they would a loud, demanding patient who always knew his rights.

Sister Doherty, the sister in charge of the men's ward at the hospital, was like the angel of death. If she saw a patient and did not think much of him, his number was up. He would rarely last more than two or three weeks. I was never sure whether she was a discerning diagnostician, unaware of the powerful primitive instinct that she had in her or whether she was such a grim, forbidding person that if she decided somebody was going to die, nobody dared contradict her.

One of the most unforgettable cases that I saw in my early days was that of a young, soft-spoken farm labourer who came in with extensive gas gangrene of his leg. He had cut his knee a couple of weeks before while pitching manure and then came into hospital, desperately ill, with this bloated, smelly leg that crackled when you touched it, and with swelling ominously going up into the lower abdomen.

He didn't complain. He stoically received any treatment that was given him. The whole hospital loved him and willed him to get better. The chances were that, at best, he would lose his leg, and at worst, he would die, with the second of the two much more likely.

I never remember the hospital so geared into action. Jack and I shared the giving of the anaesthetic as we were having to pump blood and various other substances into his veins. Henry operated, with Steve assisting him.

'If I take the leg off,' said Henry, 'it is still not going to help. It has extended to the abdomen. We will just have to keep cutting.'

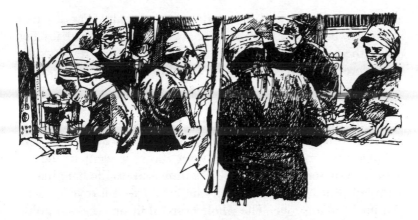

The enemies of gas gangrene are fresh air and blood. The organism that causes it lives only in dead tissue where there is no oxygen. It spreads by poisoning and killing the surrounding tissues and extends progressively as it creates the surroundings which it likes best.

We had eight hours in the theatre the first night, with Henry patiently cutting each pocket of dead tissue; cutting it away, encouraging bleeding, with the ever patient Steve swabbing and pulling retractors. The four of us, with the theatre staff, worked right on through the night. The theatre porters (who could well have gone home) stayed on just in case they could be of any use and proved invaluable, rushing further supplies of transfusion fluids and making themselves generally useful.

I had never experienced such a will to fight for a man's life being shared by a whole hospital. Every patient and nurse in the place knew about him. They all enquired how he was getting on. People forgot their own troubles and their own illnesses. This man's life suddenly became the focal point of the hospital. Nobody was going to spare himself or herself.

Eventually, at six in the morning, Henry said, 'This is all we can do for now. If I have cut the abdomen clear we will have the leg off later, and he will stand a chance.'

We took over Henry's practice duties that day so he could remain with the boy all the time but by two o'clock in the afternoon we were all back in the theatre again. The leg had improved but the gangrene was beginning to spread further across the abdominal wall. Henry continued to cut dead tissue, to explore, to clean, to swab. Steve held the fort in the practice on his own while Jack and I fought to keep this young man alive, not only from this deadly organism that was attacking him but from the terrible mutilation that Henry was having to inflict in order to try and stop the disease taking him over.

Four times more in the next three days we went to theatre with the boy semi-conscious all the time and his life hanging on a thread. But on the fourth day he began to improve, and he continued to improve. The whole hospital lit up – he was going to make it.

He had another three or four troublesome weeks in hospital and had twice to go back to the theatre. But he survived.

He kept his leg – a terribly scarred leg – but, what was much more important, he kept his life.

Six months later I saw him hobble into Outpatients, still with his gentle, pleasant smile, with no other scars from this terrible ordeal other than the knife marks on his leg. He would not be able to work on a farm any more but there were other jobs he would be able to do, and I felt that he owed his life to himself. It was his own gentle, unassuming personality which created this tremendous spirit in the hospital to get him better.

I had not appreciated before what a powerful effect the real concern of people for each other could have on their chance of survival. Stoicism was a different quality. There were some tough old men in Tadchester – hard as nails. You would see them walking about in winter without jackets – just a shirt, boots, no socks – particularly the miners from Thudrock Colliery. While I was shivering in my overcoat they seemed oblivious to the elements.

The National Health Service, whose advantages I feel always outweigh its disadvantages, offers what is called the Domiciliary Consultation Scheme. This enables me to call a specialist from the hospital (provided I can get him to come) to see patients in their own homes. This saves the patients having to trek up to the hospital feeling unwell, or sometimes from having to be admitted to hospital.

One of the physicians from Winchcombe Hospital, my old friend John Bowler, was always happy to come. John was a delightful man in his early forties. He pretended he was a frustrated general practitioner, and enjoyed entering people's homes and seeing patients in their own surroundings rather than giving brief impersonal examinations in Outpatients.

If I was worried, John would come. He got a small fee from the Health Service for his visit, but the fee was small enough to discourage many of his colleagues from rendering the same service.

The difficult people to get out on domiciliary consultations were the surgeons. Surgeons are always wealthier than physicians because they make most of their money from private operations.

There was a private nursing home in Winchcombe and two of the surgeons spent more time operating there than they did at the hospital where they were supposed to spend at least nine-elevenths of their time.

They were able to remove an appendix for £50 or do a hernia for £100, but they were reluctant to travel fifteen miles to Tadchester to see someone in their own home for a fee of £7 which could not be paid in cash and would be taxable.

With Henry away on holiday one summer, I had to call in one of the Winchcombe surgeons. It was a real battle to get him over.

It was for old Tom Barnsley who lived Up the Hill. A retired collier, Tom had intense abdominal pain. He had had it for two or three weeks before I saw him, and adamantly refused to go to hospital. It was only when he had been vomiting for forty-eight hours and had obviously become obstructed that he agreed, reluctantly, for me to get a surgeon out to see him.

The senior surgeon from Winchcombe, who was also the duty

surgeon, eventually and with poor grace agreed to come. He arrived late, and parked his Bentley outside Tom's terraced house. He examined Tom without talking to him and without even removing his overcoat.

'Yes,' he said to me, in a high nasal voice, 'we will have to operate on this man. If I do an incision here' – pointing to Tom's abdomen – 'and cut across here' – drawing with his finger tip a line from Tom's ribs to his navel – 'I should be able to resect this blockage. It sounds like an appendix adhesion to me, but I must get cutting as soon as I can. Get him over straight away.'

Tom, who had a dignity of his own, did not blanch while the dismemberment of his body was under discussion. As the surgeon turned to go, Tom, quite seriously and meaning every word, said, 'Could I make a request, sir?'

'What is it, my man?' said the surgeon, turning impatiently to him.

'I realise you are going to do all this cutting up of my stomach,' said Tom. 'Would it be possible for me to have some sort of anaesthetic?'

The surgeon stamped out of the room without answering him.

Only I had realised the genuineness of the question.

'Don't you worry, Tom,' I said. 'We will see that it doesn't hurt. I will make sure that you're fast asleep before he starts.'

'Thank you, sir,' said Tom. 'Maybe in my young days I could perhaps have put up with it, but I am getting on a bit now and it might be more than I could manage without something to deaden the pain.'

I loved Tom at that moment. I knew who I'd take with me on a tiger hunt if I had to choose between Tom and the surgeon.

Alas, all my patients were not stoical. They were outnumbered by at least ten to one by the non-stoical or even minus-stoical.

A great non-stoical was George Barrow. For some time I had been suspicious of him and felt he was getting the better of me.

He used to come periodically to the surgery with, 'It's my chest again, Doc.' He produced a most convincing cough which, he said, prevented him sleeping nights. Work, he said, was quite impossible.

I would say, 'Is there anything else?' and wait for his stock reply which was, 'Yes, my stomach's bad too, Doc. I think it's the phlegm that gets on it.'

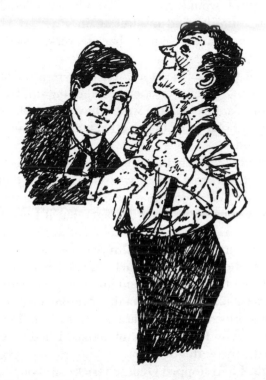

I would listen to his chest, but could find nothing. I had him X-rayed a couple of times, and the films were always clear. In spite of this he was still able to convince me of the sincerity of his story. He would be off work for three or four weeks, and then come back with a martyred expression on his face and say, 'I've still got the cough a bit, Doc, but I have to get back to work.'

I found him out eventually, one day after he had reported sick. I happened to call out into the country, at a cottage where

Jack Tomlinson – a schoolmaster – had a smallholding. Jack was repairing a shed roof to make it waterproof for the winter. And there was George Barrow working away in his overalls.

'What's the matter, George?' I said. 'I thought you were off sick.'

'I thought I would give Mr Tomlinson a hand,' he said. 'You know – until I find my feet again.'

'I'll give you a hand, George – back to work,' I said, and signed him off on the spot.

Jack then told me the story. There were a lot of run-down cottages about. Whenever one needed doing up, George – who was a man of many parts – would have a few days off sick to help restore it. He was an expert cottage restorer and was in great demand.

I was never sure whether the people whom he helped with their restorations knew that he was off sick or not. Jack obviously knew. He said that at one time George was even going to suggest to me that I came in on a percentage; that if I put him off sick while he was repairing somebody's cottage, I could have a percentage of his National Health Service money.

This time he had said to Jack, 'That friend of yours, Doc Clifford, he's a fine doctor. I went into the surgery and sat down, he took one look at me and said, "Mr Barrow, you have got the broncho-bloody-itis. You are not fit to work." So if I can't go to work, while I've time on my hands, I had better give you a hand with the cottage.'

I thought I had stopped George's tricks until one day he came into the surgery smiling, and said, 'I wonder if I could have a sick note, doctor.'

'What's the trouble, George? Chest again?'

'No, it's my hernia, doctor – it's giving me trouble.'

I looked back through George's records and found that he had had his hernia for fourteen years.

I said, 'It's a bit late in the day to come.'

'It's giving me pain, doctor, I can't work with it.'

'Very well then,' I said. 'We will fix you up to have it

operated on at the hospital. Dr Johnson is in the surgery – we'll make arrangements now.'

George's face fell a mile.

I visited him on my hospital rounds, but then I lost track of him until, about four months later, I saw him whitewashing another dilapidated cottage out in the country.

'How long have you been back at work, George?' I said.

'I'm not really back,' he said. 'This hernia, you know, never really settled down after the operation and Dr Hart said he didn't think I was quite fit to return yet, so I thought I would fill in a bit of the time painting.'

George grinned, and I tried not to. But I couldn't help smiling. We both knew he had won.

Little Miss Shepherd walked briskly into the surgery. She was a bright, twinkling seventy-five-year-old whom I saw very little of in the surgery. She lived about five miles out from Tadchester, away from the coast, in a woody area called Hart's Woodlands. She was one of those uncomplaining patients who were over-grateful for any small service you did for them. My one visit to her home to treat a very severe bronchitis was rewarded by a bottle of her specially made sloe gin being sent to the surgery for me.

Her complaint this particular morning was that she had slipped and bruised her hip. Could she have something to rub on it?

I examined her hip carefully, and tried its full range of movements. My pulling her about caused her very little pain so I prescribed some anti-inflammatory tablets and gave her some oil of wintergreen to rub in. I had learnt that Tadchester patients loved warm and smelly ointments. It was all part of the cure.

I saw her a couple of times more in the town on market day. She got a lift in with a neighbour and sat in the Pannier Market with assorted vegetables, dressed chickens, home-made chutneys and jams for sale.

I was surprised, two months after her first visit, to have her limp into the surgery, not so brisk this time, and obviously in a lot of pain.

'I am afraid my hip is getting worse, doctor,' she said. 'Do you think I've got arthritis?'

Her hip was painful on movement and I noticed that the foot of the affected side was turned out, as opposed to her good leg where the toe pointed firmly forward.

'We'd better have it X-rayed, Miss Shepherd,' I said. 'We will see just what is going on in this hip of yours.'

I got her X-rayed that morning and went to see the wet X-ray plates with the radiographer. I was appalled at what I saw. The whole of the head of the left femur had crumbled. I had missed an impacted fracture of the neck of the femur. I had heard that people could crack their hip bones and walk about on them for months, but had never seen it happen before.

Poor Miss Shepherd.

We sent her across to Winchcombe Hospital where her hip was pinned. Happily, two weeks later I saw her in Pannier Market. There was a little bit of a limp when she walked over to me, but she was as cheerful and bright as ever.

'Thank you so much for all your help, doctor. They have stuck me together again and I am fine. There are one or two little things I am sending round for you. I am so grateful.'

I cringed. This was all for a misdiagnosis on my part.

Back at the surgery were two bottles of sloe gin, a couple of chickens and a basket of assorted, scrubbed, and neatly tied vegetables.

From then on anybody who had hip pain was going to be X-rayed.

A woman holidaymaker of forty-two had slipped on a rug at home and had been given aspirin by her own doctor. When she came to me her hip was aching more because she had been swimming. She also had the foot of the affected side pointing out a bit, so I had her X-rayed: again, I found an impacted fractured neck of the femur.

She had to be sent to Winchcombe and on my half day I

went over, very pleased with myself and my brilliant diagnosis, looking forward to thanks and gratitude, especially as I was making an effort on my half day to visit this person who was far from home. Instead of gratitude I got blistering abuse for having spoilt her holiday. I was dumbfounded.

When I told my tale of woe to Steve, he smiled.

'In general practice, Bob,' he said, 'you will find that you get a lot of praise where you don't deserve it, you will get a lot of abuse when you don't deserve it. But on balance we get far more praise than we do deserve. You just have to take the rough with the smooth.'

13

Birth of a Doctor

One of the reasons I had been invited to join the Tadchester practice was that I had an additional qualification in midwifery – D.R.C.O.G. (Diploma of the Royal College of Obstetrics and Gynaecology).

Steve Maxwell was wanting to give up midwifery: he felt he had done his share. Henry, who somehow combined surgery and general practice, was making grunting noises about cutting down a bit in the area because his operating sessions were going to be increased.

I had done a year's residence in midwifery and gynaecology in London. I had also had a long-lasting and serious affair with Brenda Collins, one of the midwives there. The affair didn't increase my medical knowledge vastly, but it did teach me a lot in other directions.

I had got as far as taking Brenda home to meet my mother when she decided that one of my colleagues, who was going to specialise and was better breeched than I, was better husband material than just a potential general practitioner.

It was after the end of our affair that I took the position of Senior House Officer at Winchcombe General Hospital. From there I had gone to Tadchester armed with all the latest midwifery knowledge and techniques. I had been used to working with a back-up team of nurses, house surgeons, anaesthetists, and hospital theatre facilities. I had actually done three Caesareans on my own. When I say 'on my own', the obstetrical registrar assisted me throughout and held my hand.

I felt equal to any childbirth emergency that Tadchester might provide and preened myself on the fact that my three partners were looking to me as the specialist.

We were very badly off for midwifery facilities at Tadchester. There were no maternity beds at the hospital. A couple of miles down the road, however, was an old nursing home where the National Health Service allowed us to confine twelve patients a month. St Mary's, the nursing home, did have running water, electricity, and a resident nursing staff, but when I looked round for anaesthetic machines and the instruments and apparatus I had been used to working with, the others just laughed at me.

'You are on your own here, Bob,' said Henry. 'You pack everything in your bag: needles, stitching material, forceps – the lot.'

'What about anaesthetics?' I asked.

'Oh,' said Henry, 'one of us will come and put a drop of chloroform on for you. You will notice there is a bottle in your bag.'

My heart sank. There were no transfusion sets, no blood, no oxygen, and none of the special apparatus for reviving the new-born.

The only hospital midwifery beds were at Winchcombe, and totalled just fifteen. They had to serve an area covering a fifty-mile radius. All my partners considered it a failure to send a pregnant mother into hospital. They filled me with horrific stories of swinging on forceps and removing afterbirths from patients lying in feather beds. It all sounded terrible.

During my first delivery at St Mary's, which I was doing myself with the aid of a part-time nursing auxiliary, the Matron's spaniel wandered into the labour room, lifted his leg against the table on which I was conducting the confinement, then made a dignified exit.

This was country midwifery?

Somehow we never had any real trouble at the nursing home although we had several scares. Winchcombe Hospital, with all its sterile, aseptic wards and nurseries, was always getting infections and cross-infections. At St Mary's, in spite of the primitive conditions, we never ever had an infection.

Once a fortnight we ran an ante-natal clinic at the surgery. Nurse Plank, our district midwife, helped us with the documentation and assessment of each case. Nurse Plank was one of the pillars of the community. She was in her late fifties when I first met her. I expounded on the latest techniques and what we should be doing now rather than the old-fashioned ways they were using. She just nodded as if she had seen this all before. She was, in fact, an absolute gem. The mothers loved her.

In her thirty years in midwifery she had delivered some thousands of babies, most often on her own. She was calm and unruffled during deliveries, and never turned a hair when there were great haemorrhages or when things were not going right. I found to my chagrin that, in spite of my up-to-date knowledge, she knew a great deal more midwifery than I did. I came to rely on her so much that if I knew she wasn't going to be at a confinement, I used to get cold feet, hoping that she would be back before the baby arrived.

The vast majority of women in the town had their babies at home. To get into the nursing home you either had to have something wrong with you or be without some of the basic necessities, such as toilet facilities, electricity, and running water.

I did conduct confinements in front of open, blazing fires, with only a few small glimmering candles to supplement the firelight. On average I had three home confinements a fortnight. They could last for anything from ten minutes to two or three days, with me nipping backwards and forwards, wondering whether I should interfere and whether I was just giving up if I sent a mother into Winchcombe.

It was one of the most satisfying aspects of general practice. Pregnant mothers are one of the few groups of patients with whom a doctor can look forward to a happy ending.

Confinements I enjoyed most took place in the outlying farms that surrounded Tadchester Down the Hill. It was so much part of natural farm life – just like lambing time. Nobody would look for complications, and they very rarely occurred.

We would be sitting in the bedroom during the confinement – Nurse Plank, usually the farmer himself, and the mother in labour. There was a relaxed air about it all. The deliveries always seemed to be relatively straightforward. After delivery, they were all delighted to get some new healthy stock. There would then be a cup of tea and scones all round, or sometimes cider or sloe gin, the local speciality.

One farm confinement I didn't enjoy was when the mother began to haemorrhage profusely after the delivery of her baby. I pumped in the maximum dose of every drug I had that might have reduced the haemorrhage, blocked the bed, reassured her as best I could, sent for an ambulance and sat with her, watching her get paler and paler as the flow kept on.

At that time there were no midwifery flying squads. The ambulance always took at least an hour to arrive, and if it were summer with holiday traffic about, it might take one and a half hours to get the patient into Winchcombe Hospital.

In those days we didn't carry transfusion sets or plasma, and I had to sit there watching this young mother slowly fade away in front of me. There was nothing more I could do.

The mother must have caught some of my concern. She asked anxiously, 'Can't you do anything, doctor? I'm not going to die, am I?'

But it had gone past the time when I could reassure her. And she sensed my anxiety.

After what seemed years, the ambulance arrived with two hearty, cheery ambulance men. I have never been so pleased to see anyone. They had transfusion equipment aboard, and I was able to get a plasma transfusion going. Slowly her pulse, which had dropped to a flicker, began to pick up and was easier to detect. She had lost so much blood that the bleeding had stopped. I thought she couldn't have had any left.

I rode with her in the ambulance to Winchcombe, checking her pulse every few minutes. She just held her own till she got there. She was whisked to the theatre and in twenty-four hours she was sitting up, bright as a button, feeding her baby as if nothing had happened.

I felt at least fifty years older.

*　　*　　*

I still had not taken part in any real heroics, the sort my partners bragged about, where they had had to put their feet on the bed to help them pull out babies with forceps. But my turn was to come ...

I had one young expectant mother at home who obviously had a huge baby, and who was not making progress. Although I had helped babies out with the small forceps we used for low forceps deliveries, I had never put on the great big ones or had to use any degree of force to help with the extraction.

I had to ring Jack and Henry to come and give me a hand – we were obviously in for a picnic!

Jack anaesthetised her by dropping a mixture of chloroform and ether on to the gauze mask over her face. Henry prowled round, grunting and unconcerned, while I, the specialist in midwifery, sweated. I was going to have to prove my worth.

'Hurry up,' said Henry, taking his ear from the woman's stomach. 'The little one in here is beginning to get fed up with it all.'

I managed with great difficulty to get the forceps applied to the baby's head. This was a huge one.

Then I started to pull.

'Hang on!' cried Henry. 'I'll hold her arms.'

So, with Henry pulling one end and me pulling the other, the poor woman was almost being dragged in two. Nothing was moving. I just didn't know what to do.

'Come on, lad,' said Henry. 'If you don't do something we're going to lose the baby.'

132

I put my foot on the end of the bed for leverage, and pulled. The baby's head came through, tearing the tissues round it. The bed, which was raised off the ground by four wooden blocks, came off its blocks and crashed down on the floor, making a terrible din.

The poor girl's husband, who was sitting below, came running up the stairs at the noise, wondering what could have possibly happened to his precious one, and was just in time to see the rest of the baby appear.

It was a bit blue in the face but after a few slaps by Nurse Plank it breathed and cried lustily.

I had joined the club!

'Well done, lad,' said Henry. 'She would have lost this baby if it hadn't been for you.'

This particular mother and father actually lived some miles away and were not our patients. They had come to Tadchester to have the baby in the home of the girl's parents. So, after the delivery, I lost sight of them.

Some years later I saw them again, walking through the town. The little boy must have been about seven years old. I noticed that he had a walking iron on one leg. It looked as if he had had polio.

'What has happened to the young man?' I asked. 'Did he have an accident?'

'No,' said his mother, blushing. 'They say it was the result of a birth injury.'

I remembered how proud I had been, leg levered against the bed, tugging for all I was worth to get this baby out. But, of course, if I hadn't he would never have seen the light of day.

Happily, as obstetric care has improved and more hospital beds have become available at Winchcombe, we don't nowadays have to deal with this heroic type of midwifery.

My next forceps birth was quite different.

I had been called by Jack to give him a hand at a gypsy encampment. They had sent for him after labour had started – she had never been seen by a doctor during her pregnancy.

She was obviously in obstructed labour. Jack said he would rather give the anaesthetic and let me try and pull the baby out.

It was a tiny caravan with a bunk bed. There was only just room for me to work at the foot of the bunk. Applying the forceps was not too difficult, and after just a moderate traction pull the baby came out quite easily and all was well.

I cut and tied the cord. We had not been able to locate Nurse Plank for this one. I picked up the baby to put it in its cot before I tackled the afterbirth. Forgetting the confining strictures of this particular labour room, I took one step backwards and fell through the half-door of the caravan down the steps, clutching the newly born baby to my chest. I had never felt so foolish, and the baby didn't like it at all.

There were six or seven Romany men sitting round the camp fire watching all this with interest. As I tried to get up from the grass, at the same time trying with one hand to keep the baby clear of the ground, one of them strolled over.

'You a bit new to this game then, doctor?' he said, grinning. I could have kicked him.

People seemed to have babies in all sorts of places. Although the vast majority did have them at home or in the nursing home, I was called to deliver in buses, taxis, garden sheds, fields, and once in the back row of the cinema.

But I wasn't always there in time.

One morning I had a call at two o'clock. I heard a gruff voice say, 'Is that you, doctor?'

'Yes,' I said.

'This is George Hobbs here, of ...' went on the gruff voice, and he named a hamlet ten miles from our surgery.

'Would you come and see the wife straight away?' he asked.

'What's the matter?' I enquired.

'I think it's a maternity case,' said George.

'What do you mean?' I said. 'You *think* it's a maternity case. Has your wife seen a doctor recently?'

'No,' he said. 'I think it's a maternity case.'

'Is your wife in labour?'

'I think it's a maternity case,' said the gruff voice, and George rang off.

I got out of bed, grumbling, and set out to find the cottage of Mr Hobbs. This was a new type of call. I had never had anybody before call me in any doubt about whether the case was a maternity one or not. They were usually sure it was – or, like Mrs Richards whom we shall meet later, certain it wasn't.

I eventually found the isolated cottage, and a six-foot, thickset, unshaven farm labourer let me in. He was completely unconcerned. We walked through a downstairs room where there was one chair, one table, and no other furniture.

'Come upstairs, doctor,' he said.

I followed him upstairs. In one of the filthiest rooms imaginable was a bed in which a woman was lying with a baby between her knees, with the cord still attached to the afterbirth, and the afterbirth still firmly in the mother.

On one side of the room were four children lying asleep on the floor with a pile of blankets on top of them. Through another door I saw a further room with three more children sleeping, covered with a similar pile, either lying directly on the boards or with a thin mattress beneath them. Even at this time I occasionally found conditions like these.

I immediately set to and completed the delivery of this now lustily bellowing child. It was completely hopeless to try and nurse it at home, so I sent the husband off for Nurse Plank. Ringing up from the nearest farm I fixed up to get the wife into St Mary's for a few days. There was not even a towel, a sheet or anything to dry your hands on in the house. I had to tie off the umbilical cord with a piece of string I found on the floor.

I also rang the Welfare Officer, who said she would come and give a hand with the other children. I then came back to the house, where the children were beginning to stir. There seemed to be no food in the place but nobody seemed terribly bothered.

Nurse Plank followed me in and started to bustle around. By this time it was seven o'clock in the morning. I refused the tea proffered in a dirty cup, and wearily packed my bag and made for the car.

George leant over the gate watching me go. He seemed dirtier and more unshaven than ever. He grinned, or rather leered, knowingly at me. 'Well, doctor, I were right – it were a maternity case, weren't it?'

Every doctor I meet thinks that his patients, and particularly his midwifery patients, are stranger and more complicated than any other doctor's patients, and can hardly wait for someone to finish telling him of their own particular hazard or mishap before he is telling them his own. Though I would not claim that the complications, sites of delivery and excitement of my own cases are second to none, I feel that I could hold my own in most company.

I have had patients who have sworn they did not know they were pregnant or in actual fact didn't know they were.

Mrs Richards, a woman aged about fifty, who lived near the cemetery, sent for me one night with 'ramping' abdominal pain. On examining her stomach I noticed how large her abdomen was and that she was having regular rhythmic contractions.

'When did you last see a doctor?' I asked.

'Oh,' she said, 'I saw Dr Hart when I started the change of life eight months ago. I was putting on weight and he gave me some slimming tablets, but now I've got this terrible "ramping" abdominal pain.'

I said, 'I hate to break this news to you so suddenly, but you are going to have a baby in a few minutes.'

'Oh, good God!' she said. 'It can't be true. My daughter expects a baby any time now. I could be a grandmother by the end of the week!'

... Nellie Block could have been described as the young man's comforter in the village. Poor Nellie was a bit simple, and quite unable to refuse the approaches of any man. Over a few years I delivered her of five children of mixed fatherhood.

Her last pregnancy was a bit different. Usually she turned up at about six months with a swollen tummy and an ashamed look. This time she came in with the right statistics but looking triumphant. As she entered I said, 'Well, Nellie, where do you want to have the baby this time?'

'Oh, there's no baby,' said Nellie with a superior air.

'Are you sure?' I said.

'Oh, yes,' she answered, and fished out a dirty piece of paper from her pocket. 'The young man that I'm going with has given me a certificate to say that he's only got one kidney, so I know I'm not pregnant.'

Events were to prove her wrong.

By far my most enjoyable confinement ever was when Lily Biggs, the wife of Jack Biggs, the local scoutmaster, had her baby at home.

Jack was a great handyman and had rigged up every conceivable aid to make the whole process easier. This included a television set at the foot of the bed.

The climax of her labour came just as Freddy Trueman was beginning to get through the Australian wickets in the England versus Australia Test on the television. I couldn't see the screen properly from the side of the bed so Lily said, 'You could hop up next to me, doctor, until the pains come.' So, between pains, I lay on the bed with Lily admiring the batting. During pains, I crouched at the bedside, encouraging her.

'Come on, Lily,' I said. 'Let's see if you can push this new young wolf cub out before the end of the next over.'

Young Freddy Statham Biggs grew up to be a great credit to his parents.

14

Come Quickly, Doctor

I was called out of my morning surgery by Henry Johnson, my surgical partner, to come and give a patient a whiff for a difficult obstetric case. This was a typical unruffle-able Henry. A 'whiff' meant anaesthetising patients with chloroform, which had hazards of its own and meant something had really gone wrong.

I leapt into my car with the anaesthetic bag and shot up to the council houses that covered the top of Up the Hill. I was some time finding number 47, which was the number Henry had given me, as it lay back from the main row of houses in a cul-de-sac.

Obstetric emergencies in the home were always nightmares to me. I had been so used to all the comforts of a maternity hospital. I shuddered at the primitive way things were carried out in the country.

I entered a rather dimly lit room to find a pale, thin woman with an absolutely huge abdomen lying on a bed in obstructed labour, with Nurse Plank fussing round, and Henry, in a detached way, looking out of the window.

Henry was one of the tallest, thinnest men one could wish to meet. When clothed and gowned, with his rubber gloves on, he looked like some willowy ghost.

'Got a breech here, Bob lad,' said Henry. (This meant that the baby was arriving feet first instead of head first.)

This would have worried me to death, but not Henry: nothing seemed to perturb him.

'If you could put her to sleep, I will bring the legs out.'

Henry was marvellous practically, but I was never quite too sure about his ante-natalling. Normally one would have expected to have found that the baby was in a breech position before this stage.

I got out my cotton mask and chloroform bottle, added some ether to the chloroform and started to pour drops on to the mask over the patient's face. I hated giving anaesthetics like this. One had so little control. There were no aspirators to suck out mucus from the patient's mouth, or proper airways. The patient often went into spasm trying to breathe these noxious vapours and there was no preparation for anaesthesia. For all I knew this patient had a stomach full of plum pudding and might vomit any minute. But there was no alternative other than to get on with it.

As soon as she was well under, Henry, who was so capable with his hands, delivered the legs of the baby which were holding things up, and in a couple of minutes the baby, who looked about six pounds in weight, emerged.

'Well done, Bob,' said Henry, 'you can bring her round now.'

I looked at the huge stomach that I had noticed when I first came in; its shape did not seem to have altered at all.

'Are you sure we have finished, Henry?' I asked.

'Oh, the afterbirth will come all right,' said Henry. 'Get her round.'

'I am not thinking about the afterbirth,' I replied. 'She still looks as if she is loaded.'

Henry reluctantly put his hand to her abdomen.

'Oh my God, lad,' he exclaimed, 'you are right. There is another one here.'

In a short while, after a few more efforts, a second baby appeared head first this time. The patient had had five previous pregnancies and once this baby's head had seen the light of day, it shot out to join its five-minute-old brother.

139

'Bless my soul,' said Henry. 'Twins! That is a surprise.'

I looked down at the abdomen. It had decreased in size, but not as much as I expected.

'You wouldn't like to check once more would you, Henry?' I said. 'It still looks a bit big to me.'

'Rubbish, lad,' he said. 'She is bound to have a big placenta to feed these two. Give her some ergometrine.'

He casually palpated the stomach and started to take his gown and gloves off.

As ordered, I gave the injection of ergometrine. This is a drug that makes the womb contract. It reduces the chances of bleeding after childbirth, and although it can trap the placenta in the womb, it is often expeditious in helping it come early.

A minute after I had given the injection, the woman gave a cry, and I looked down just in time to see a third baby being literally shot out of her. The ergometrine was certainly working.

'I thought there might be three,' said Henry. 'Tip him up a bit, he looks a bit blue.'

I wondered what effect the catapulting into the world of this little fellow would have on his future psyche. Nurse Plank, who was almost as unruffled as Henry usually, lost her cool. She now had three babies to bathe, and had to find somewhere to put them, as well as enough linen, nappies, nightdresses, etc., for this treble chance. She scurried about, muttering under her breath.

'Thank you, Dr Johnson,' said the patient as soon as she came round from the anaesthetic, 'you were marvellous.'

'Don't think about it,' said Henry. 'The place to have your baby is at home, no need to go into hospital.'

It was all so incredible, I thought I might have a nervous breakdown. Somehow all the catastrophes that might have happened had not; we had three healthy babies where we thought there was only going to be one, and we had a healthy mum. It always seemed to be this way with Henry; he did not appear to worry that things might go wrong, and somehow things never did go wrong.

The mother of the new three was a Mrs Sarah Wilkins – she now had eight children to contend with. She was a thin, emaciated woman, who seemed to carry all the cares of the world. As she explained to me, when some time later I had to visit one of the triplets, 'It's when my husband gets his gym shoes on, we always click.' She went on eventually to finish up with eleven children.

Mrs Wilkins was not the only one of my patients who was given bizarre signs that her cohabital duties were about to start. Mrs Merchant (married for the second time at the age of sixty, having been widowed in her mid-fifties) married a retired farmer from Canada who had returned to his mother country to spend his last days in Tadchester. When she married him she believed him to be sixty-five – in actual fact, he was eighty-seven. His physical prowess, however, was in no way related to his age. Mrs Merchant said that she had had to put up with more physical demands for her services from her new octogenarian husband than she had had from her first husband (a sailor) some forty years previously. 'Doctor,' she said, 'he is just wearing me down. If he starts drumming his fingers on the table after supper, it is always a sign that I am for it. Couldn't you put something in his medicine?'

Returning my anaesthetic bag to the surgery after the triplets, I was pounced on by Gladys. 'An urgent call, Doctor Bob. There is a child in a caravan at Sanford-on-Sea who has difficulty in breathing.'

I grabbed my case and made what speed I could to the permanent caravan park at Sanford-on-Sea.

All the caravans had different names. There was no system of numbers and 'Kosicot', the name I had been given, could have been any of the one hundred or so scattered round the field. It was winter and only a handful were occupied at this time of the year.

I drove round for a while, trying to pick up the name, then got

141

out of the car to ask more specific directions from a caravan that looked as if it might be occupied.

As soon as I had turned my engine off and climbed out of my car, I got my directions. From three caravans down from the one I stopped at I could hear what sounded like the barking of a seal.

I rushed to the caravan. There were two young, anguished parents walking up and down, wringing their hands, and a baby girl of about eighteen months lying on her back in a bunk, blue in the face, fighting for her breath, and with each intake of breath making this harsh barking sound that I had heard when I got out of my car.

'Doctor,' said the mother, 'she was well until an hour ago. Do something. Please do something. She can't breathe. I think she is dying.'

The baby looked awful. I hated croup. It is caused by swelling usually due to infection of the lining of the main breathing tube (trachea). Sometimes the only remedy is a tracheotomy, which means opening a hole in the throat and inserting a tube. I had never had to do one and hoped that this wasn't going to be my first.

I picked up the baby, cleaned the mucus from her mouth with my handkerchief, and cradled her in my arms, with her head down.

'Put the kettle on!' I snapped. 'I want some steam.'

The mother, all thumbs, seemed to take an age to fill the kettle and put it on the gas. I waited impatiently for the kettle to boil, cradling the baby. Her breathing had become a little easier since I had been holding her. I think babies do pick up their parents' apprehension and someone from outside, appearing to be in control of the situation (although I am sure I felt as nervous as the parents), somehow gets through and reassures them.

When the kettle had boiled I told the mother to pour the water into a bowl. Then, arranging a towel round the baby's head with the bottom end encompassing the edges of the bowl, I held the baby's face over the rising steam.

142

In minutes the noisy breathing had stopped. In ten minutes the baby was happily sucking a bottle as if nothing had happened. Mother, father and I sat drinking a cup of tea made with the remnants of the water from the boiling kettle.

'It's wonderful,' said the mother. 'I thought we were going to lose her.'

I went over the baby's chest with my stethoscope and prescribed an antibiotic. I instructed the parents on how to give steam if the baby's breathing became difficult again, and suggested that they keep the atmosphere in the caravan steamy for a while by keeping the kettle on the boil.

I hated dealing with croup. This time steam had worked like magic, but it wasn't always so effective, and I had had nightmare ambulance journeys to hospitals with gasping babies, wondering whether we would get there in time. Somehow we always had.

After my second emergency I returned to the surgery a bit weary. I knew there was bound to be a third before the day was finished ... and I did not have long to wait. I had just seen one patient, a very smartly dressed Swedish lady visitor who came in as a temporary resident. The style and cut of her clothes gave the impression that money was not a problem, but she had filled in a card to have free treatment on the National Health Service, and had waited her turn with the other patients. She sat down in my surgery and in the most delightful broken English said, 'Doctorh, I passed zis snake zis morning; do you sink zere iz zomething in ze food?'

She opened her handbag and pulled out a Kleenex tissue which contained one of the largest roundworms I had ever seen. It certainly did not match her coat and gloves, and was certainly not her style.

I explained to her that this sort of infestation could be picked up from unwashed vegetables and prescribed some pills and medicine that would rid her of any possible relatives of this offending beast. I wondered which snake in the grass had managed to infect her thus.

She was followed in by Gladys with the inevitable third

143

emergency. 'Sorry about this, Doctor Bob, but someone has collapsed in the barber's shop Up the Hill. There are not any more details.'

I shot across the bridge to the barber's shop, to find the 'emergency' fully recovered and having the other half of his shave. He had been nicked on his left cheek and fainted when he saw some of the blood on the barber's towel. He had been tipped back in the chair until he came round, then the operation had continued. Everybody was apologetic, but I was happier when an emergency turned out to be a false alarm rather than a terrible medical drama.

Charlie Lang ran the barber's shop Up the Hill with his son Nigel. Charlie was one of the old school – a tough lad, taciturn, a real Tadchesterian, with about five hundred relatives in the town. He knew exactly what he wanted and what he was going to do. He liked his pint, and had obviously been a bit of a lad because, in his history, there was a report from his Merchant Navy discharge record that he had had venereal disease. This left some scarring in his waterworks which held up the flow of urine from the body. This meant that, to have a clear flow of water, every so often Charlie would have to go up to the hospital and Henry would have to dilate his water passage with some probes.

When you are dealing with waterworks in men you have to be very careful that you do not introduce infection when you are dilating the urethra (tube) in the penis, or passing a catheter (drainage tube). Any slackness in technique could result in the introduction of infection, causing cystitis and inflammation of the kidneys.

Charlie had to attend regularly every three months for dilatation. He did this for many years and then, suddenly, stopped. We thought he had gone away as neither of my partners nor I were called on for our professional services. Reluctantly, however, one day he did have to come to the surgery. He had a tooth abscess, didn't want to go to the dentist, and wanted something to clear it up. One of his characteristics of dress was that he wore an old, battered, brown bowler. I felt sure that he even wore it in bed because he had it on every time that I saw him; he wore it when he was cutting hair, and he was wearing it as he showed me a mouthful of dirty, septic fangs in the surgery.

'How are the waterworks, Charlie?' I asked. 'I see you haven't been up for some time.'

'Oh, I manage it myself now,' said Charlie. 'I couldn't be bothered to keep on going to the hospital.'

This puzzled me. I could see no way that Charlie could manage it himself.

'How do you mean,' I said, 'you manage it yourself?'

'Well,' he said, 'I went to an auction sale at a doctor's house in Winchcombe and bought myself a catheter. Whenever I want to pass water, I just slip it in my Jimmy Riddler.'

'And,' I said, 'what happens if you want to go now?'

'Well, I would just pop into the toilet and slip it in,' said Charlie. As he said this, he removed his hat and there, inside the hat, wrapped in a dirty piece of newspaper, was an old gum elastic male catheter.

Charlie had obviously watched Henry Johnson carefully when he was passing his probes. He must have been catheterising himself several times a day with a dirty, infected catheter and somehow the Good Lord (and it could only have been Him) was keeping the germs away.

'Does your water ever burn, or do you feel unwell?' I asked Charlie.

'I did a bit at first,' said Charlie, 'but I have no bother now.'

With that he picked up his prescription and made a hurried exit.

I talked to Henry and Steve about it the next morning at coffee. I could not believe that anybody could defy all our careful aseptic techniques and get away with it. But Steve said Charlie wasn't the only person administering his own therapy; there were one or two other elderly patients who catheterised themselves and there existed, in fact, fancy silver catheters that one could carry in one's breast pocket like a fountain pen and slip in and turn on the tap as required.

Henry said he thought these old boys must initially have had infections but were too tough to worry about them, eventually building up a resistance to the germs they pushed in several times a day, becoming immune to them.

I never thought much of Charlie's hair-dressing salon – it was dirty, scruffy and very unhygienic. I resolved that under no circumstances would I ever go there for a haircut, for who knows, I might not be as resistant to Charlie's germs as he was.

15

Thick Ears in the Sunset

One of the things that I had not taken into account in coming into general practice was the extra-medical or para-medical duties that would be thrust upon me.

The Forward Medical Aid Unit was the first group to obtain my services. Being flattered that people should approach me for my extra-medical skills, I foolishly took on virtually everything I was asked to do. I became Hon. Medical Officer to the Tadchester Boxing Club. This meant attending all their boxing tournaments, listening to small boys' chests and pronouncing them fit to go into the ring and half batter each other to death.

I had boxed as a medical student and shared the apprehension of these white-faced little boys as they kept running off to spend pennies before climbing into the ring to do damage to their friends.

My own boxing career was a very chequered one. I had, in all, about a dozen fights for the hospital, and at one stage was awarded the name of 'One-Round Clifford'. I was usually in the ring for just one round – but this did not mean that I destroyed all my opponents. In actual fact it worked out at exactly 50–50. Half the time I destroyed them. The other half, they destroyed *me*.

When I first went to the hospital, having come straight out

of the coal mines, I thought that with long and hard practice I might eventually make the hospital boxing team. Two weeks later, I was boxing against a dentist from Guy's Hospital at the Coldstream Hall before a crowd of several thousand.

It was a painful experience. My opponent was almost as unskilled as I was, and although we could attack, our defences were terrible and we solidly battered each other over three rounds before he was given the verdict on points.

My opponent later achieved fame in the Press at the time of his society marriage. The day before his wedding he had had to have an anti-typhoid injection, and he arrived at the church feeling very poorly. When he joined his bride at the altar steps he was visibly swaying on his feet. The vicar, a teetotaller and a leading man in the Temperance Society, immediately assumed he was drunk, and refused to marry them.

I found that the only qualification you had to have to get into a university or hospital boxing team was to be foolish enough to be willing to take part. So few people take up the sport that even Oxford and Cambridge Universities sometimes are unable to turn out a full team. It is the quickest way of achieving notoriety in sport and the easiest way of winning a Blue.

We had in our hospital the undefeated flyweight champion of London University for five years. He achieved this without a scar as, in fact, he didn't have a single fight. There was nobody of his weight who would volunteer to fight. Only once was he in danger of losing his title. This occurred when we found he was two pounds above his weight limit. We forcibly administered castor oil and in a matter of three hours had him back on the scale below the limit and earning two points for our team.

My second fight was against Oxford University at Oxford. There was some sort of matching of people of equal ability and I was to fight their secretary who was, according to them, about my standard. When I got there I found that (a) he was a welterweight – I was a lightweight – and (b) I had had one, unsuccessful, fight and he was in the Ceylon Olympic Games Team.

I lasted just under a minute in the ring before they carried me out.

My friend George Potts, who had come along for the ride, agreed to fight – only because his opponent in the match was a young man who had never fought for the university before. What they had not mentioned was that he was the Royal Navy's middleweight champion, George lasted either three seconds more or three seconds less than I did. We both claimed the longer distance.

Against Cambridge University I somehow got my thumb in the eye of my opponent in the first round. I watched the eye swelling during the round and prayed that it would close completely in the interval.

My prayers were answered. The referee came over and stopped the fight. I had my first victory. It was thumbs up for me!

On one occasion I found myself in Dublin fighting against Trinity College for Guy's Hospital, who had borrowed me for the occasion. It was Trinity Week and I had a glimpse of what university life used to be like before the war. The sports meetings, rowing, beautifully dressed ladies, and men in frock coats and top hats. There was even a picture of me in the Irish *Tatler* being rubbed down by Mat Wells before my excursion in the ring.

I climbed into the ring with some trepidation but after a few seconds realised my opponent was even worse than I was. I got him into a corner to finish him off, then suddenly I found myself in a dark room, with water pouring down from above on top of me. I couldn't understand it. Was I dead? What had happened?

This is a gap in my life that I have never remembered. My friends told me afterwards that, as I pinned my opponent in the corner, he shut his eyes and swung in despair with his right, nearly knocking my head off. I vomited for two days after this brief encounter and my closest friends say I have never been the same since. The saddest part was that the great steaks that I brought back from Ireland (the meat ration in England was then about a shilling's worth a week) I was too ill to eat.

It was at this same match that the Guy's heavyweight lost his unbeaten record. He was a huge brute of a man, and the small Irishman who had been put up as a sacrifice stood trembling in his corner before the bell rang for the first round. As his elephantine opponent approached him, he ducked to miss the oncoming blow. The Guy's champion caught his arm in the ropes, dislocated his shoulder, and the Irishman was declared the winner.

Of my twelve fights I won six and lost six. I have a prize possession – a cutting from the *Evening Standard* describing one match against Cambridge University where it said the most punishing bout of the evening was when R. D. Clifford fought G. D. Lockhurst. It went on, 'R. D. Clifford, after surviving severe punishment, rallied in the last round, to beat his opponent on points.'

This just about sums up my boxing career.

Giving a helping hand to sports I did not mind. I did enjoy them and felt that I had to put something back into the games I had taken part in. The activities that I found most tedious were lecturing to groups like the Women's Institute, Church-women's Guild, and Mothers' Union. Tadchester seemed to have at least one of these organisations on every street corner. I became an expert at judging fancy egg and comical potato competitions and had to make judgments on flower arrangements, needlework, cake baking and a dozen other such competitive indoor sports.

One disastrous day I foolishly agreed to judge a baby show.

I started the day thinking that my decision would have to be made between the six babies that were presented to me, and spent over an hour deliberating. It was then that I discovered there were another eighty-three to see.

My judging went on for hours, past feeding times, resulting in expeditions being sent out for powdered milk and an exhibition of mass breast feeding in the reserved tent. This resulted in the curate having a nervous breakdown – hearing so many babies crying, he walked into the tent to see if he could help and, for the first time, really found himself in the bosom of his parish.

My final judgment caused joy only to the parents of the baby who was awarded the prize. Three of our patients with babies transferred to another practice and I made several mortal enemies. How could anybody possibly think any baby was better than their Jane or Susie?

My main love as a student was for rugby and I soon became a Vice-President of the Tadchester Club. If I had not played rugby there was little doubt that I would have qualified a year earlier. Rugby was an extremely important part of medical school life: in fact, when I first went to my hospital they unashamedly offered rugby scholarships to boys who had the necessary academic qualifications. This meant that when we played against other hospitals in the Hospital Rugby Cup Competition we were always greeted with cries of 'Come on the Professionals!'

I tried one or two games when I first got to Tadchester but general practice was very demanding and I could never train or get properly fit. When I came out of one game with a painful knee, Steve pointed out very gently that a one-legged G.P couldn't climb the stairs of country cottages as well as a two-legged one. I got the message and, reluctantly, hung up my boots.

I became an ardent supporter of Tadchester and was conscientious in my duties as Vice-President, helping behind the bar, attending committee meetings, and acting as Hon. Medical Officer.

Tadchester were a good little team, with ambitions to break into the big time. The only really first-class side they played were Winchcombe, the local giants. Winchcombe really played a different league. They had everything to lose in this particular match, whereas Tadchester had everything to gain.

Eric and I watched a lot of rugby together, and we muffled up on a cold, wet day to watch this annual battle.

The Winchcombe men seemed twice the size of the Tadchester players. Two threequarters with foreign-sounding names I had never seen play before. It was a good spirited game but Tadchester were completely overwhelmed, losing by thirty points to three. The main architects of the victory were these two foreign threequarter backs who turned out to be French and were working for a year with a Winchcombe electronics firm. They ran and handled so much better than their British counterparts. Drinking in the bar afterwards with them took me back to my own rugby-playing days as a student and my first French rugby tour.

* * *

I shall never forget the first French tour. And I shall never know how I survived it.

We had assembled at Victoria Station the day after a very hectic Cornish tour. I had played three games in three days, the third game being abandoned in the middle of a torrential downpour.

We were to go by boat and train to Paris, stay the night, then by train to three games in the Rhône Valley area, train back, a further night in Paris, and then back to London. It sounded marvellous.

We were going to play some of the best French rugby sides. I had some doubts when I looked at the motley collection of people who were arriving to make up our party. For some years the hospital side, with half a dozen current Internationals in their strength, had been one of the best in the country. By some means these stars had just qualified, making the Cornish tour their rugby swan song. From now on the hospital was going to have to rely on lesser mortals like myself.

Combined with the withdrawal of these experts, the French tour itself coincided with the hospital inter-medical examinations. It had been impossible to raise the invited twenty-eight players from the first three hospital sides, so the vacant places had been offered to people who either deserved to go, like the jovial captain of the 'B' XV and the rugby club social secretary, who never really played rugger but arranged the rugby dance on which the finances of the club depended, or some who didn't deserve to go, like the beer-drinking layabouts from the extra 'B' and 'C' XVs.

There was one character I couldn't place. I assumed he must be somebody's relative. He claimed to be a trainee manager from the Savoy Hotel. How he came to be included in the party I never knew.

We had a calm crossing but one or two of us, still feeling the effects of the Cornish tour and the rained-off game, felt sick.

We arrived in Paris with a night to spend before we went on to Lyons. We had been told that tea, coffee and old suits fetched good money on the black market in Paris, and we came well supplied.

We had a hectic night in Paris, first selling our tea, coffee and suits on the black market, then on to pubs, night clubs and, eventually, the Bal Tabarin, from which we were finally evicted at four in the morning. There was little money left when we staggered to the train at 8.00 a.m. the next day.

We had an interminable journey to Lyons, where we entertained the French by wandering down the corridors, singing the filthiest English rugby songs.

From Lyons we got another train to Tarrare which was the venue of our first match. Arriving in the middle of the afternoon we were whisked straight from the station to a champagne reception at the hotel, and then to a dance that went on until three in the morning.

I had learnt two French expressions before I came away – *Tu a des yeux bleu*, and *Voulez-vous me donner le plaisir de cette danse?* Both served me well during the evening.

We were the first English side to play in this town since the war and they really did their utmost with their hospitality.

153

We were playing a local representative side the next day, and everyone assured us how easy the game would be. This was the equivalent of a first division soccer team playing one of the southern league teams.

The morning following the dance we had a Civic Reception. This was followed by a tour round a silk factory where we were wined and given champagne until an hour before we played.

We played on a sun-baked pitch in the evening against this local enthusiastic side. We had not put our strongest team out, although I am not sure what our strongest side was. If we had played all twenty-eight of the party I doubt if we would have been as good as the normal team.

There was an impressive start. The French kicked off a high, long kick for their forwards to follow up. Our full-back from the 'B' XV, the most sociable chap, stood there like a rock waiting for the ball to be caught and safely disposed of. If he had been able to wear his glasses there is no doubt he would have been a first-class rugby player, but without them he was as blind as a bat. As he stood there, arms open, firmly fixed to the spot, the ball bounced about twenty yards behind him for a French forward to pick up and score a try.

The French, realising then that we had a blind full-back, exploited this for the rest of the game, and we lost 12–11. They all nudged each other, and said, 'These English, they keep their cards up their sleeves, wait till they play the big game tomorrow.'

Again that night they treated us to another dance and champagne party. The captain of the 'B' XV, celebrating his success, sat at a table quietly on his own with thirteen empty champagne bottles in front of him.

The next day we played Lyons at the Lyons Olympic Stadium. Before we started, a band of white-gauntleted gendarmes paraded round the pitch playing martial music. An immaculately turned-out French team trotted on to the pitch to the cheers of the crowd, and then we trotted on. It was the first time

I had really taken a look at us as a group from, shall I say, an aesthetic point of view.

These were the days of clothes rationing and rugby clothes were the last thing for which coupons could be spared. We had played in Cornwall, our kit was still wet and filthy from the mud bath of the rained-off game. Nobody had cleaned his boots, we were caked with mud and really looked scruffy.

I was better dressed than most. As a spare shirt, I had taken an old green one (we were playing in blue) that my grandfather used to wear for playing soccer; it had a lace-up neck, to which I had laboriously sewn a semi-stiff white collar.

We lost to Lyons 25–3, but we weren't disgraced. They were pleased to win, and it was quite a good game. It was always best on a French tour to just lose each game; you then can be assured that the social side of the tour will be marvellous.

We had a dinner in Lyons with the Lyons Club, which ended by our captain doing a naked Zulu dance on the table during which he accidentally poured a glass of wine over the head of Madame la France who had been the head of the Resistance for that area and was the guest of honour at the dinner. She must have wondered what she had achieved with all her heroic efforts.

She had helped to oust the Germans from her country only to have them replaced by a naked South African pouring wine over her.

We had a scrum down in the hall against Lyons, during which all the glasses were broken – then, drunken and singing, we were led to the bus that was to take us to our next destination.

The bus journey was a nightmare. We had been playing rugby and drinking and travelling now for as long as I could remember. People were being sick, people were fighting, people were being obstreperous.

We arrived at our next destination where we were being boarded out with families, instead of being put up at an hotel. There were rows of cars and pleasantly smiling French people to welcome their allies and liberators. The only way to describe our leaving the bus was to say that we spewed forth from it. Immediately the waiting hosts saw us, half the cars disappeared without taking anybody. Several of the boys lay down in the Square, quite unconscious, and half of us, instead of sleeping the night in comfortable French beds, eventually finished up roughing it in a barn.

The next day, after one more Civic Reception, we were to play this town which had a very good side. The previous year the hospital side, with all stars present, had come back from 17–10 at half time to win 20–17.

We were in pretty desperate straits by now and agreed to play the substitutes. This was about as un-British as one could be in rugby, but our substitutes served us manfully. Every one of the whole twenty-eight of the party came on to the pitch at least once. Our waiter, and I am quite certain he wasn't the trainee manager from the Savoy Hotel, came on five different times in five different positions. The captain of the 'B' XV played in the forwards, where he didn't have to see the ball and played much better. The social secretary came on as wing forward in the first half. After tripping everybody up and getting in everybody's way, he committed his worst crime at half time: throwing his orange peel off the field, he hit our only mobile threequarters in the eye with it and disabled him for the rest of the game.

We had all taken Dexadrine tablets to help liven our performance but at half-time we were down 30–0. The French, remembering the come-back of the year before, waited hopefully. After half-time our Dexadrine began to work. We were up. We stormed the French and we got seven points in as many minutes – a dropped goal and a try. This was the stuff they wanted.

The crowd was on its feet, but in a few minutes our Dexadrine had worn off and we were eventually beaten 45–7. We played so badly that this town didn't invite another English team for five years. There was the inevitable Ball and Banquet after the game. By some booking mistake we had no seats back to Paris the next day, and we had to stand, crammed between the toilets of the two coaches. Another night in Paris and then home.

I was flat out in bed for four days when I got back. When I did finally emerge and ring round my fellow players to see how many were still alive, I found that I was the first to surface.

I went on several French tours after this, but never again to the Rhône Valley – they wouldn't look at us.

I never forgot my first French rugby tour – and obviously the French never forgot the English.

16

Swings and Roundabouts

My duties in the general practice at Tadchester were to be split up between the ordinary general practice duties such as surgery, visits, midwifery, etc., and my work at the hospital. There I doubled with Jack Hart for emergency anaesthetics, and kept a day to day check on patients of mine in the wards, some of whom might be under the overall care of one of the consultant physicians from Winchcombe.

Most of the Winchcombe consultants held outpatients' clinics at Tadchester Hospital and would come over and see cases that we were worried about or felt needed extra special care.

In addition to this I had to take a rota share of doing casualty duty at the hospital.

The casualty sister at Tadchester Hospital was a short, plump, fierce Welsh lady called, strangely, Sister Jones. What she lacked in height, she made up for in ferocity: many a Saturday night drunk was completely sobered by the sharpness of her tongue. She was a hard, unsympathetic, efficient woman who kept herself very much as a private person, someone you could work with for a hundred years without ever knowing. She was very uncommunicative, but completely reliable. If she called you for an emergency, you went. There was no argument. Her assessment of priorities was always exact, and while a doctor was treating patients she would stand over him, fussing, trying to tell him what to do as if she knew much better – which, of course, she probably did.

I was terrified of her, would ask her nodded approval before I would start any procedure, and never had the strength or courage to contradict her. She had a succession of staff and pupil nurses to work for her, whose lives were made a complete misery. They were nagged from dawn till dusk and were never given a word of praise when they did something well or efficiently.

When Sister Jones was not on duty the atmosphere in Casualty was quite different. The nurses smiled, got on with the jobs capably and did not seem to need this all-seeing dragon to keep them up to the mark.

The main casualty duties were in the summer when Tadchester was jammed with holidaymakers. There were two holiday camps at Sanford-on-Sea, numerous caravan sites tucked away Down the Hill, one or two small hotels in the town and larger ones dotted in a radius of five or six miles around, some with their own beaches reached by pathways through the cliffs.

Holiday visitors had special categories of ailments of their own. There would be a whole string of patients suffering from jellyfish stings when the tide had thrown up more than its usual collection of these transparent menaces.

Food poisoning was always rife in the summer and on one occasion both the two holiday camps were stricken, with everybody wanting to sue the management, holidays ruined, and terrified chefs fleeing the area for their lives.

The fairground that came in late August, as well as producing numerous cuts and scrapes from people falling on and off the roundabouts or sticking legs outside dodgem cars, usually produced a crop of venereal diseases, and a couple of weeks after it had gone one or two shamefaced young men and ladies of the town would come and present themselves with pain in a very embarrassing area.

Occasionally some of the fairground attendants would come for treatment for this same condition. It was obviously a hazard of their trade, and there was no doubt that the young ladies of Tadchester were fascinated by these romantic men of the road and could easily be induced to give their all.

The Casualty Department seemed to be filled from the beginning of the summer to its end: the slackening of casualties was an indication that winter would soon be upon us.

We were unable to persuade holidaymakers to visit the surgery for their wasp stings, sun burns, and small cuts and grazes – hospital was the place for them.

This was unfortunate for us, as one of the strange anomalies of the National Health Service was that we did our casualty work as a charity. We reaped the vast sum of £10 per year for all our hours of sweated labour, whereas if these hordes of patients had visited us at the surgery they would have been signed up as temporary residents under our G.P. umbrella and we would have received £1 for every one we saw.

We had a continual battle with the Authorities to make it financially right for our service, but there was no loophole by which they could pay us, even if they had been willing. Rather than give up this service, we soldiered on for next to nothing.

Henry philosophised: 'It's swings and roundabouts; we must keep on with it;' whereas Jack said, 'Swings have always made me sick; I would much rather stick to roundabouts.' Swings or roundabouts, casualty duty gave a division of work which for me was invaluable, for I was able to continue to practise many of the skills that I had learnt as a house surgeon.

There were tedious procedures like getting beads out of noses, foreign bodies out of eyes and ears, but there were rewards like splinting broken arms and legs and a great deal of stitching up of wounds. Stitching practice was very important: one's skill as a seamstress determined whether a badly cut face would be scarred or not.

The summer holiday traffic brought innumerable road accidents. During the season we had to battle to save the lives of dozens of horribly maimed and mutilated victims, in situations where all our skill and resources had to be used just to keep life flickering until more sophisticated equipment could be brought into play. Having to keep on our toes for these emergencies made better doctors of us all.

Sometimes we were called from Casualty to attend to accidents themselves. One I never forget was on the main road leading to Sanford-on-Sea where a family car, packed with mother, father and two children, with all the paraphernalia of food, blankets and stoves, had crashed head on with a young couple driving an MG sports car. The MG was a complete write-off, with the young couple both dead, with broken necks.

The scene in the family car was chaotic. Its older vintage had made it more robust than the sports car and it had not disintegrated in the same way on impact. When I arrived the father was struggling out of the front seat with blood pouring down his face, the two children screaming on the back seat, and the mother unconscious, with both legs trapped and bleeding under the compressed dashboard.

We managed to get both children out, one of whom had a broken leg. Borrowing a sledge hammer, I got into the back of the car and smashed open the door by the mother, applied tourniquets round both her legs and then, with the help of a crowbar, levered up the dashboard, dragged her out and into the waiting ambulance.

It was a night's lost sleep for all of us.

The mother had broken both legs and had suffered severe lacerations. Henry, Jack and I were in the theatre for two hours with her.

The husband and children had to wait for their treatment until we had patched up the mother. The husband had lacerations to the scalp and a broken arm. One child had a broken leg and the other a broken arm.

I imagined them setting off happily for their holiday, to have it destroyed in one blinding, flashing moment, the same moment that took the lives of the young couple, out for an evening's drive. Instead of a summer by the sea this family spent some weeks in Tadchester Hospital, the mother being transferred to

Winchcombe after a few days for more specialised orthopaedic treatment.

*　　*　　*

Like other branches of medicine in Tadchester, Casualty had its collection of curios.

One day I was called urgently because a holidaymaker had gone into labour in the Casualty Ward. When I got to the hospital she was stretched out on the small operating table in the casualty theatre with the baby's head just beginning to emerge.

The staff nurse – Sister was off duty – said this was a girl from Bristol who wasn't due for a month and had suddenly gone into labour. There was a fifteen-year-old youth standing nervously beside the screen in a corner of the room whom I assumed was her brother.

Looking at the emerging baby, I thought the girl must have been wrong about her dates: this baby certainly was not premature. It was a good eight-and-a-half pounder, and she had a fair old push to get it out.

There was something familiar about the girl's face but it did not register at the time. When the baby had been safely delivered and the umbilical cord tied, the staff nurse took the baby to be bathed while a student nurse and I waited for the afterbirth to come.

At this moment the girl on the table said, 'Can I go now, please?' and tried to get up. If we had not restrained her, she would have been up and out of the Casualty Department in a flash, with the cord trailing and the afterbirth still inside her.

We tried various manoeuvres to get the afterbirth, but after an hour it was firmly stuck. As she wasn't bleeding, I decided to send her to the obstetric unit at Winchcombe Hospital to have it dealt with.

We rang for an ambulance and packed her off. Just as she was about to leave, the fifteen-year-old-boy asked if he could go with her. I still assumed that he was her brother, so reluctantly gave my permission, and they were whisked away.

Next day I learnt the full story from the girl's mother, whom I knew quite well.

The girl's face *had* been familiar after all, and the fifteen-year-old boy was no brother: he was the baby's father. And this wasn't the first child they had had between them – it was the second. I remembered clearly an account of their first mating when, apparently, he was thirteen-and-a-half and she was fifteen-and-a-half, and he had got his way with her by offering her a bottle of ginger beer. Their union was blessed and subsequently adopted.

I asked the mother had she noticed that her daughter was pregnant, and she said no. Her daughter had worn a wide flared skirt with a high belt, and she had had no idea about the increased pounds and swelling tummy underneath, and in fact the girl had been working as a cleaner at the hospital a few weeks previously.

She decided to keep this baby rather than give it away like the first. The parents of both sides got together and decided, as there was strong or even duplicated evidence of a long and lasting relationship between these two young people, they should be given the opportunity to marry when the boy became sixteen.

'Not on your life,' said the girl. 'I wouldn't marry him for anything. We're only friends.'

*　　*　　*

I enjoyed my hospital work and got to know most of the staff well. Whenever some bright-eyed nurse took my fancy and I tried for a cuddle in the dark room of the X-ray department I was always put off with, 'You will have to wait for Christmas.'

Preparations for Christmas in the medical fraternity in Tadchester started in early November. There were draw tickets to be bought from the Sister of each ward of the hospital. They all vied with each other to have the best show and I had, as

163

early as October, been invited to carve the turkey on the children's ward on Christmas Day.

The hospital was only one of several medical institutions that were competing for our services over the festive season. St Mary's Maternity Home put their claim in. Steve looked after a home for mentally defective children. It was called a 'home'; in fact it was more like a hospital, with 150 patients, and although it was called 'for children' some of the inhabitants were in their seventies and eighties, having spent all their lives in institutional care. I enjoyed the odd occasions I had to visit the home. They were mostly mongols, who were friendly and affectionate and led happy, trouble-free lives, with other people doing all their worrying for them. They had an extremely high standard of care there and, whatever age, all remained children. It was like a house full of Peter Pans, with excitement when anything interrupted the routine, like trips to the seaside or holidays away.

High up Up the Hill was a small isolation hospital which, since the virtual disappearance of tuberculosis, was hardly ever used but had to keep a staff in case there was an outbreak of some virulent infectious disease. The staff there had more time than any to prepare for Christmas.

Last, but not least, there was the Old People's Home or Hospital. This was the old workhouse that had been converted into a home for the care of the aged and although a couple of wards there were full with people whose bodies were still alive but whose minds had died some time ago, most of the patients or residents were ambulant and Christmas was the highlight of their year. It was a time when relatives who tended to neglect them most often turned up and when relatives living away, coming home for Christmas, had their only opportunity of visiting Gran or Grandad.

As Christmas approached, my mantelpiece became filled with invitations to all these various hospital or near-hospital functions, and by mid-November I saw that I had every night booked from 21st December till 2nd January. They must have had a very good medical fixture secretary somewhere as none of the dates clashed.

It looked as if I was in for the most hectic Christmas ever. I had had a few hospital Christmases as a hospital resident, which had been hilarious, and all very drunken. I was obviously going to have to pace myself over this fortnight as there would no doubt be people requiring my medical services during this time, particularly if they had to follow the same party schedule as I did.

My first four pre-hospital parties were similar, in fact almost identical, as exactly the same people were at each party. They all wore exactly the same clothes at each function and apart from slight variations of drinks and eats, it would have been difficult to distinguish one party from another.

Eventually Christmas Eve arrived, with the traditional carol singing round the hospital. It looked most moving. The nurses wore their capes turned inside out so that the scarlet lining showed, and carried candles. An assembly of friends and hospital staff joined to swell the volume of carols as we did a circuit round the wards. This was the highlight of the year for the hospital pharmacist, as he walked round accompanying the singers on his piano accordion.

We must have totalled about seventy in number and, when in full voice, made all the hospital timbers rattle as we limbered up with our First Noel in the courtyard. It was all for the patients' benefit. However, because we tried to get as many patients home for Christmas as possible, there were only about a dozen patients left in the whole 150 beds. Most of these were pretty poorly, one or two in oxygen tents.

We set off trooping round the wards. It was a delightful and moving sight, with the lights turned down, illuminated Christmas trees in each ward, and the flickering of the nurses' candles silhouetting their white headgear. In the women's ward the two ladies in oxygen tents must have been very apprehensive of all the naked candle flames slipping past them. The two remaining ladies fit enough to breathe without artificial aid were so overcome by this moving scene that they sat up in bed with tears streaming down their faces.

We toured all the wards – women's medical, women's surgical, men's medical, men's surgical – and there was no doubt that the patients who were well enough to appreciate it absolutely loved it.

I was happy that they had managed to clear all patients out of the children's ward, which was up a flight of stairs. I thought that they might have been a bit overwhelmed by the noise because, as we got more confident with our carols, so our volume tended to increase. But tradition was tradition, and although there was nobody in the children's ward we solemnly, all seventy of us, walked up the stairs, circled the ward in full voice, and then walked down to be received by Matron with coffee, mince pies and Christmas cake.

Christmas had begun.

Christmas Day proved to be an absolute nightmare. Every department of the hospital vied for one's attention. Steve had warned me: 'You miss having a drink in one department of one hospital and you will be blacked for the whole of the year.'

The nurses in each ward dressed up the doctor who was to be their particular carver. I was to be Batman and had to struggle into some black tights, a red jersey and face mask. This was to be my costume for the day. A glance in the mirror showed me that since I had stopped playing rugby my waistline would have shamed Batman. The tightness of my tights showed to the world at large that I was fairly well endowed in one part of my muscular anatomy that they probably had not had a glimpse of before. I now knew how ballet dancers felt.

I started off on my pre-lunch tour of the hospital. Not only did it mean a drink in each department, but it meant embracing every nurse in every department. By the way some of them clung on I felt they were all trying to get rid of a year's inhibitions in a day.

I had a sherry on women's medical, a sherry on women's surgical, a sherry on men's medical, a sherry on men's surgical.

By now my mask was half covered with lipstick and my tights had begun to sag.

I had a sherry in dispensary, a sherry with the operating theatre staff, a sherry in Outpatients, and a sherry in Casualty.

I then staggered up to the children's ward and did my carving for the staff there. Two children had been admitted in the early morning, both with moderate burns, and were not at all interested in the riotous goings on.

I had finished my carving by one o'clock and then set out, with sherry coming out of my ears, to do my rounds of the other medical and semi-medical places. My tights were no protection from the bitterly cold weather and I received derisive cheers as I drove round the town in my Batman's outfit.

I had a sherry and a mince pie at St Mary's Maternity Home, I had a sherry at the Children's Home, I had a sherry at the Old People's Home and then, finally, my last duty sherry at the Isolation Hospital, who were offended that I wouldn't stay and have a second glass with them. 'Nobody spends any time here,' they grumbled.

By now it was half-past three in the afternoon, and I could hardly see to drive. I eventually made it to the Harts', where I was having Christmas dinner, got out of my Batman outfit into warm, respectable clothing, and set to work to remove the lipstick from my face.

I staggered downstairs. 'What will you have to drink?' said Jean Hart, smiling. 'I know you need something to pick you up.'

I groaned, sat in a chair, and fell fast asleep.

Fortunately the Harts had become adjusted to hospital Christmases and Christmas dinner was not until eight, by which time I had begun to come round from my over-indulgence.

The post-Christmas week was slightly different. This was the dancing week. There was the Tadchester Hospital Dance, the St Mary's Nursing Home Dance, the Old People's Home Dance, the Isolation Hospital Dance, and the Children's Home Dance. Most of them were related to raising some funds for one charity or another but, again, apart from a few guests who had come over from Winchcombe, the assembled company was exactly the same as it had been at the four cocktail parties the previous week.

During my first Christmas in Tadchester I came to realise that I had a strange facial characteristic that made me look as if I were a man who preferred whisky to any other drink. Even in the hospital wards where sherry was the proffered refreshment, there was always a wink from whoever was in charge and a, 'Don't worry, doctor, I saved a bit of the hard stuff for you.'

I had to fight to stick to the same type of beverage, as I actually preferred sherry to whisky, which I don't really like at all. The impression that I gave in the hospital was reflected in the gifts from my grateful patients. They had all been generous when I first came into practice. Christmas gave them a great opportunity to redouble their efforts. Although I was given a turkey, Christmas pudding, Christmas cake, sweets, and a couple of pheasants, the main bulk of my gifts were bottles of whisky, ranging from quarter, half and pint bottles to what must have been two-litre bottles. There was enough whisky in my flat to have happily bathed in it.

At every visit I made over the Christmas holiday there was usually a glass of whisky thrust into my hand, and to have refused it would have caused great offence. I would down it as quickly as I could, and be off, but of course I would go on to my next visit smelling of whisky. So, whatever drink there was about to be offered would be hastily exchanged for half a tumblerful of this terrible amber fluid.

This routine went on day after day and I had begun to lose track of time and place and found it terribly difficult to concentrate on my work.

It is indeed, a terrible physical affliction – to have the face of a whisky drinker!

The last engagement on the calendar was the Grand Ball on New Year's Eve. This was the Tadchester Hospital Ball, held in Tadchester Town Hall, and was different from the other hospital functions in that all the local civic dignitaries had been invited as well as most of the consultants and hospital management staff from Winchcombe Hospital.

It was a very good Ball, so I'm told. I was in such an alcoholic blur that I couldn't really remember what happened. Somehow I got through it without disgracing myself too much.

For some time afterwards, one or two ladies complimented me on excelling myself at the Ball. I had no idea what they were talking about, but as each finished her conversation with a knowing wink I had obviously been close to a few fates worse than death.

New Year's Eve was on Friday evening and, thank God, I was able to get to bed at three o'clock on the Saturday morning.

I knew I could not take much of this.

I fell sound asleep and woke up to find myself in the dark. I was puzzled because my watch showed it was six o'clock. I had to turn on the radio to discover that I had slept through till six p.m. Sunday.

I resolved, of course, never to take alcohol again.

By Monday morning I had begun to feel better, and went off to work with a good heart. The surgery was light, people were not yet well enough to come and see their doctors.

I set off to have a look at my patients in hospital, wondering what scenes of destruction would greet me there, but it was as if somebody had waved a magic wand. All the Christmas decorations had gone, the wards were full.

There was hustle and bustle. The familiarity of Christmas had disappeared. We were back at work again.

Christmas was over.

17

Friends and Neighbours

Among the inhabitants of Tadchester I found some great characters and made some very good friends. There were the young group that I went around with – Kevin and Janice, Frank and Primrose, Joe and Lee, and the ever-faithful Eric.

We fished, swam and supported the rugby club together, and spent some of our most delightful evenings Seine-net fishing. Our mishaps were perhaps the greatest part of the fun. Once, I remember, we fished all night and caught nothing. Only when we got back did we realise that there was a hole in the back of the net through which a medium-sized shark could have swum.

On one occasion we joined with another net and swept from both ends of the beach. It was a big tide and there seemed to be miles of sand to cross. Janice and Primrose were pulling our box of fish, which got heavier and heavier. We could see them occasionally in the darkness as we came out of the sea.

When we were walking back to the car Janice said, 'This sled is running easily now. You wouldn't think we had all that fish in it.'

A quick flash of the torch showed that they had been pulling the box on its side for the last half mile. We had to trek back looking for sledge marks, trying to pick out the fish that were beginning to blend into the beach. Frank, to whom fishing was almost a religion, said some unprintable words which certainly weren't religious.

My favourite Tadchester character was Old Bob Barker, who had the secondhand bookshop by the slipway at Sanford-on-Sea. He was in his eighties when I first met him, and was the gentlest and wisest man I ever remember.

For many years Old Bob had had a large bookshop in Tadchester, which became a meeting place for writers. He had a room at the back where he held small literary lunches, and he helped several famous authors take their first steps into the pages of public literature. When it all became a bit too much, he sold his big shop and had this small secondhand bookshop at the water's edge. He and his daughter would always take time and trouble in finding or searching through catalogues for books for customers. They charged very little for these services. Their enjoyment was in doing things for people, and they were happy just to make a reasonable living from their work. Book orders came from all over the world, and this rather shabby little shop and its gentle proprietor were quite famous.

I used to spend hours poring over the old books on the shelves. After some time I was invited to have tea with the great man himself and eventually a great friendship grew up between us. Although Old Bob was a non-smoker, he saw to it that in his desk there was always a box of my favourite cigars, with one ready for me when I joined him for our cup of tea. It became a ritual that I would sneak away for an hour a week with Old Bob. I would listen to his tales of the people of the area, the lords and ladies, the tradesmen, the craftsmen and other types of people who went to make up the community.

Between us we used to set the world aright and we both looked forward to this hour of stolen time each week. He used to be desperately disappointed if, for some reason, I failed to make it.

He was very conscious of his growing years and his frailty. 'All I want to do now, Bob,' he said, 'is to slip quietly away. I am tired and old and I have done my share of living. It would be nice just to float away one night.'

I wasn't Old Bob's doctor; he preferred me as a friend. Jack

171

Hart looked after him for many years and always coped with his medical requirements.

Jack found that Old Bob had some waterworks trouble and would need a prostatectomy. It was a great blow. Old Bob hated the thought of it – hospitals, operations, pain, strangers, and away from his beloved bookshop.

I went to see him for our tea and cigar a week before he went into hospital.

'You know,' he said, with a twinkle in his eye, 'I have kept on saying for so long how much I would like to slip peacefully away. Now there is a chance of it happening, I have suddenly remembered an awful lot of things I still want to do.'

He survived his operation and lived on for several more years. He had been the parish church organist for many years, had a great love of music and many friends in the music world. In his eighty-fifth year the BBC recorded him and presented him as a portrait character of the Somerset coast.

When he died, he left a gap that has never been filled. He was a wise counsellor, the gentlest of men, and the greatest of friends. Since he died, whenever something nice happens to me, I think that somehow, somewhere, Old Bob Barker has had a hand in it.

He inspired in me some yearnings to do some writing myself, and in his will left me a beautiful old bound volume of *Chamber's Book of Words*.

Two other elderly people I looked upon as friends were the two Miss Emmersons – Sophie and Elsie. They lived in a semi-detached house in Park Lane, separated from the river by the park, where they could watch the children playing on the swings and slides and keep a close eye on the Council gardener, as they more or less regarded the flower beds in the park as their property. They would say, 'Our dahlias are doing well,' or 'What do you think of our chrysanthemums?' and I would be meant to look, not round their tiny garden but across to the huge flower beds in the park.

Both had been brought up as ladies, but were now in reduced

circumstances. They lived in this little house on what must have been a small income compared with their earlier days. They described some of the houses they had lived and stayed in, the balls and banquets they had attended, and the young toffs who had sought their hand.

The contents of the house bore witness to their former glories. They had the most beautiful china and silver and some lovely old furniture. Although they did not now have the income to live in the style they had been used to, they kept their gentility and manners. We became, I thought, firm friends.

They were both frail and needed check-ups from time to time and were particularly plagued by winter coughs and colds. Sophie, the elder sister, was the more dominant one and twice the size of the bird-like Elsie.

This was a visit that I couldn't get away from without having a cup of tea, and a cup of tea was not just a cup sitting on your lap. If the doctor called it was served at a table from a silver teapot, with the best bone china, scones and home-made cake. I could rarely get away in an hour and they just wouldn't have understood it if I had tried to explain how many other people I had to see that day.

They preserved their standards and I admired them and looked forward to my visits. They didn't gossip, were not malicious, and they gave me an understanding of a gracious world that I knew nothing about.

One day Elsie complained that she had begun to get pain in her lower leg if she walked any distance. If she stopped walking, the pain would go, but as soon as she had walked a further distance it would come again. It meant that if she was out in Tadchester she had to stop after every few shops and pretend to be looking in the window.

I examined her leg and found it a bit cold. The pulses were difficult to feel. She obviously had poor arterial circulation of that limb.

'Well, doctor,' said Sophie, 'what is the matter with Elsie?'

'Miss Emmerson,' I said, 'she is suffering from a condition

called intermittent claudication. I will have to get her something to help her circulation.'

This was a day on which I was in a hurry, and didn't have time to explain it more carefully.

The next time they were ill they sent for my senior partner, Steve Maxwell. They had become such regulars of mine that I thought it was a mistake, but Gladys confirmed that they definitely wanted Dr Maxwell. I assumed that they must have thought I was on holiday, and when Steve came back I asked him how the leg was.

He said that there had been no mention of the leg. Miss Sophie had bronchitis. They had made no comment about my treatment or my visits to them.

I racked my brains to try and think of some way I might have offended or upset them. It always hurt me when patients changed from me to one of my partners. (I always seemed to understand it if one of my partners' patients came to me.) And the Emmersons changing really upset me – we had been such good friends.

The same pattern went on for several months. Steve was summoned whenever the sisters were ill; my services were never mentioned and I was never asked for.

One day Steve called me into his surgery, pretending to look grim but hardly able to stop himself laughing.

'I have had to see Miss Elsie Emmerson today,' he said. 'She is complaining of a pain in her leg on walking. I believe that is what you treated her for. What did you tell them was wrong?'

'I told them she obviously had poor arterial circulation and was suffering from intermittent claudication.'

Steve rocked back in his chair.

'Do you know what they *think* you said?'

'No,' I replied, puzzled.

'Intermittent fornication. Get out of that one!'

I realised that things between myself and the Emmersons would never be the same again. Steve tried to explain to them this medical term, but I was not to be forgiven for quite a while.

I think that my misheard diagnosis struck home deeply. Perhaps between the grand balls and banquets they had attended, escorted by the gentry, the toffs and Army officers – perhaps on some occasions, with the blinds drawn or in some secluded hotel – there had been a few moments of intermittent fornication. Perhaps poor Miss Elsie thought I had read her mind. She thought her past was catching up with her.

It was far too delicate a subject to try to explain the misunderstanding. So many people think that doctors are like God and that, simply by looking at their patients, they can tell exactly what they are thinking and what they have been doing. But if Miss Elsie only knew. To see her there in her flat-heeled shoes, her long black dress, sparse grey hair and row of pearls, barely making the journey round the room, the last thing I would ever accuse her of would be fornication, intermittent or otherwise.

But eventually I was forgiven. In Miss Sophie's will two years later – and it was a very meagre will – she had left me £50 for my services to herself and her sister. She had left Steve Maxwell nothing. I did wonder whether she thought this was hush money for me to keep this guilty secret safe.

One of the penalties of helping people recover from their illnesses was that, as a reward, I would be asked to dine with them. I would be asked in such a way that there was no possible chance of escape. Like, 'Can you name a night in the next two months that you will come and have a meal?'

Though I had sweated blood to get them better, the probability was that I did not like them very much (it always seemed to be so in this type of case). I now had to face giving up a precious evening and sharing their company while they wined and dined me.

On their part it was a type of inverted snobbery. Once I had agreed to eat with them, I was on social terms and it was as if they had evened the score. I had saved their lives, they had accepted me into their house as an equal and forced an unwanted meal on me. From then on they would assume that our doctor/patient relationship was different. They would start calling me by my first name. It was a great social fillip, for example, to ring the surgery and ask for Bob Clifford as opposed to Dr Clifford.

This was the case with the de Wyrebocks. Mrs de Wyrebock was certainly anxious to level the score. A gold-embossed invitation card was sent to me, inviting me to dine with them. Pencilled on the back was, 'A dinner jacket, please.' This was to put me in my place, to show that everybody else would obviously know what to wear, but an ignorant peasant like myself would most likely turn up in a tweed jacket with leather elbow patches.

I dreaded the thought of this dinner, but it was impossible to refuse it.

I arrived at the house, to be shown in by the butler. Apart from Marjorie de Wyrebock, who was my own age, the other ten who were assembled looked as if they had all been dusted and brought out of museums.

To my great surprise the company was quite delightful. They were all old men and women who had led adventurous and full lives. These were the fit, or should I say once-fit, who feature as the survival of the fittest. I heard reminiscences of places that I had read and dreamt about. Afghan frontier expeditions. Malaya. The Boxer rebellion in China. The slaughter of the Great War when they had lost most of their friends. I did not have to speak: I just sat back and listened to these delightful old gallants and the stories they had to tell.

Even Mrs de Wyrebock was gracious and pleasant to me. The ladies did not leave us when the port was passed round. I think they were all too old and stiff to get up from their chairs, or were limited in the number of up and down movements they could make in a day.

When the port had gone round for the last time, a few of the poor old codgers were dozing in their chairs. Mrs de Wyrebock said, 'I am sure you two young people would like

176

some fresh air. Marjorie, why don't you show Dr Clifford round the vinery?'

It was only when I got up from my chair that I realised how good an evening I had had. I was full to the brim with sherry, port and wine. I had been entranced by the tales that I had heard. I was full of love for my fellow men. Even Marjorie

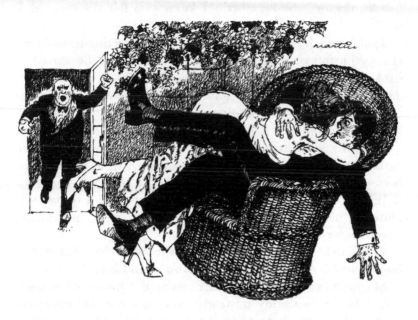

de Wyrebock, who was advancing towards me, looked quite attractive. Seen through an alcoholic haze, her teeth seemed to have shortened, and the bosom that was peeping out of her dress was certainly not unattractive. Her riding calves, which were one of her most prominent features, were hidden from view by her long dress.

She took my arm, probably to steady me, and we wove our way towards the vinery.

When we entered this large glass-walled room I nearly passed out. It was hot and humid; I was back in one of the Malayan jungle stories I had just heard.

There were double basket chairs round the room. Scattered on tables were copies of *The Tatler*, *Vogue*, and *Country Life*.

I had to sit down quickly because the room was reeling. I made for the nearest double basket chair, with Marjorie still on my arm, and dropped into it. Marjorie came down on top of me.

'Oh, doctor,' she breathed. 'I knew you felt the same as I did!'

Two horsey lips, stoutly reinforced by supporting teeth, were clamped firmly on my mouth. With her free hand she started to stroke my hair. I think 'groom' would be a better word to describe her action, and I began to sympathise with her ponies.

I must say that she didn't taste too bad and, as somehow her lips covered her incisors, I was in no fear of laceration.

With the wine and good spirits of the evening I got a bit carried away. I responded to her grooming by what I suppose in horsey circles would be called 'stroking her withers'.

Just as I had begun to raise my sights and explore her plunging neckline, the vinery door crashed open. In stormed Commander de Wyrebock.

'Gad, sir!' he shouted. 'Is this the way you repay my hospitality? I should be grateful if you would leave!'

Marjorie began to adjust her dress as if I had tried to rape her. I had to walk my unsteady way past the still occupied dining table (nobody had had the strength to move yet), collect my shabby raincoat from among the twill jackets on the hallstand under the disdainful glare of the butler, creep out of the front door, and drive myself home.

I must say my recollection of Marjorie wasn't too bad, but after getting back to my flat and having a few sobering cups of coffee, I realised how fortunate I had been to escape. Another half hour of Marjorie's uninhibitedness and it could have been a shotgun wedding. Mrs de Wyrebock had won after all. She could now send for one of my partners as, with reason, she wouldn't have that 'damned new young doctor' in her house.

I did think of putting an empty sausage skin in my thank-you letter for the dinner, but thought better of it. You can't win them all – and this had been really nearer to a draw than a dead loss.

18

After the Ball

Janice and Kevin Bird had invited Eric and myself to make up a party with two potential brides to go to the Tadchester Carnival Ball. The two ladies were New Zealanders, distant cousins of Janice. Janice was always trying to marry me off, but her idea of a desirable catch never quite tallied with mine, and I had only just got over pining for my London midwife, Brenda Collins.

When I first met Brenda she had been a young probationer, coming from a home of poor circumstances in the north. I was one of the first boys that she had been out with, and when I first met her she was untidy, badly dressed, and shy, but underneath her untidiness she had a rare beauty. She had long, shoulder length, blonde hair which she twisted into plaits and piled on top of her head when she was working. She had the most beautiful aquiline face, and perfect white teeth. I was happy to take her to her first dance, help her buy her first ball gown, and watch her grow in confidence and stature under the shelter of my company.

We were inseparable and went boating on the Thames at weekends. I took her home to meet mother. Strangely, mother and she never quite got on. Brenda always carried a chip on her shoulder and, having spent so much of her life as a Have-not, she had determined that she was going to be one of the Haves.

As her confidence grew, so did her choice of clothes. She paid much more attention to her hair, and she changed from being a frightened little probationer until she was without a doubt the best looking nurse of her year.

These were days when I was in my first year of clinical studies as a student. We were both penniless but our joy was in each other's company.

Until the time I qualified we spent our holidays together, most often camping. In our third year of camping Brenda, who had now become quite a sophisticated city girl, looked wistfully at the large hotels near the camp site and asked, 'How long before you take me to those?'

We could only see each other intermittently during the first year after I had qualified, and she went off to do her midwifery. We wrote practically every day and, by writing often enough, never seemed apart. I accepted, when we met, that she would be a bit different. She had to find to some extent her own way in life, and she did go to parties and dances without me. I only had one night a week off and I couldn't expect her to sit in every evening.

We met up together in the same hospital again where she was now a midwife and I was the obstetric house officer. She urged me to specialise, as most of my friends were doing, but I was set on going into general practice, which I felt I was best equipped for.

Brenda hated the idea of being a general practitioner's wife, tied to telephones, part of a small community. She grew more and more attracted to the bright lights, and she was increasingly being squired by Roger de Silva, one of the obstetric registrars, who was destined for Harley Street and was already partly equipped with a Bentley and a great deal of family money behind him.

It all came to a head when he asked Brenda to join a party hiring a yacht in the Mediterranean. We had bitter arguments about it, but she was determined to go.

181

I gave her an ultimatum, that if she did go it was all over between us.

Brenda did go, and she was engaged to Roger when she came back.

I kept out of her way as much as I could, heartbroken, to the end of my year's obstetrics. Then I applied for a mixed house job at Winchcombe Hospital which was in the area that I hoped to practise. I had at last got her out of my system – I hoped – and I wondered what the evening would bring.

*   *   *

Eric and I fortified ourselves a bit too long and too late before going to Kevin's. We had dulled our inhibitions sufficiently to cope with both the exotic and the just plain awful.

We arrived at Kevin's late, apologising that we had had trouble with the car. Kevin smelt my breath and said, 'Yes, I can see that. It is something to do with your fuel injection system.'

The girls were twins and could only be distinguished by the small scar that Jennifer (the older twin by half an hour) had on her right cheek. Jennifer was to be mine for the evening, and Eric had to settle for her sister, Laura.

It was obviously another bad match. I didn't fancy either of them. They were both tall, full-busted girls and, by the way they grabbed our hands on introduction, eager for the fray.

We had a drink with Kevin and Janice and then the six of us set off for the Ball.

It was packed. Everybody who was anybody was there.

We fought our way through the crowd to the bar, waving and shouting good cheer to our friends. I could see Frank and Primrose, Joe and Lee, but the noise was so great I couldn't hear what they were shouting across the room to us.

We got ourselves settled by the bar and Jennifer (who must have been over-filled with gin by Kevin before the Ball) started becoming amorous, pressing one of her great bosoms into my shoulder and stroking the back of my neck with the hand that wasn't holding her, yet one more, gin. She insisted on dragging me on to the floor for a dance and almost raped me in front of my patients.

'Bob,' she said, 'we are hitch-hiking round Europe next month. If you have got any holiday due, why don't you join us? You can share my hike tent – there is plenty of room for both of us and Laura likes sleeping out in the open anyway.'

This was going to be a frightful evening.

I fought my way back to the bar. There was only one thing to do – blot out the evening with alcohol.

My third pint was almost knocked out of my hand by the clashing of cymbals and the smash of a drum. I turned, to see the spotlights fixed on the stage and there, emerging from what used to be the old orchestra pit, in all her glory – skin-fitting deep purple dress, presumably to match her nipples, and plunging neckline that was no encumbrance to her physical charms was – Oh! my God – Gwendoline Jacobs, the Carnival Queen. I had forgotten all about it.

The M.C., Mike Thomas, Secretary of the Rugby Club, came on to present Gwendoline, who played her part, gently undulating from side to side on the stage. The Coltz XV who were sipping their shandies at the back of the stage nearly flipped their minds.

After Gwendoline had been suitably crowned and presented with a large bouquet of flowers, Mike Thomas then announced that the Carnival Queen would now start the Ball rolling with a ladies' invitation/excuse-me dance; the first man to dance with her would be her King for the night.

Gwendoline stood on the stage, sniffing the air like a foxhound. I ducked my head, trying to hide behind Jennifer's left bosom. Surely to God it wasn't going to be me. I remembered that Gwendoline was fairly determined when I examined her for her medical. I didn't look round. The bosom was soft and if I leant against it with my right ear there was room between it and its right counterpart for me to sip my pint of beer.

The room became silent. I suddenly became conscious of an overpowering smell of cheap scent. Then Gwendoline's voice.

'Doctor, will you give me the pleasure of this dance?'

There was no escape.

We had to do an exhibition dance round the floor with Gwendoline stuck to me like a limpet. Her nipples pierced my rib cage like two steel spikes. I prayed for somebody to come and excuse me.

Jennifer's embrace was like a pygmy's compared with that of Gwendoline's.

All the time we danced Gwendoline was muttering in my ear.

'Give way to your impulses, doctor. Live. We may all be dead tomorrow. I have got a caravan in Skegness for a weekend in a fortnight's time. Why not come and join me? I promise I won't tell anyone.'

I suddenly heard a horsey voice say, 'Excuse me', and a hand clutched my shoulder like a vice. I was literally torn from Gwendoline, with Gwendoline falling back looking as if she could commit murder.

I turned to face my saviour and nearly scalped myself on a row of flashing buck teeth. It was Marjorie de Wyrebock!

Whereas Gwendoline had clung to me like a limpet, Marjorie rode me as if she were a stallion. She had one hand firmly pressed to the lower part of my back, somehow pushing me up under her saddle area, and half carried me round the room.

'Doctor,' she said, 'we are going on a cruise in a few weeks' time. Mothah finds she has booked an extra cabin by mistake. What about joining us, eh? Needn't cost you a penny. At one or two places we are stopping there is some damned good riding.'

By now the floor had filled with other dancers and was so packed that I was pushed even further into Marjorie's embrace. I could have sworn that she was gripping me with her knees and managing to walk me round at the same time.

I became conscious of a small, sweet voice, persistently saying, 'Excuse me. Excuse me.'

184

Deliverance at last!

I brought my head up quickly and accidentally hit Marjorie's bottom jaw, causing her to drop me as both rows of her flashing teeth stuck firmly into her tongue.

I turned round to greet my rescuer and there, looking as lovely as I have ever seen her, was my faithless midwife, Brenda Collins.

She twined round me, cheek against mine, and we were moving smoothly round the floor as we used to a year ago. It seemed we had never stopped.

'Oh, darling Bob,' she said, 'at last I have come to my senses. It just didn't work without you. I am starting at Winchcombe next week. I had to be near you. Couldn't we start again?'

At this moment it all became too much. The after-game booze, the gins at Kevin's, and the pints since, ganged up together and decided to leave me, and with an 'Oh, I am so sorry dear,' I was sick all over Brenda's sequin dress.

I don't remember any more of the dance. Kevin and Eric somehow got me home. They said, when they had got me sufficiently conscious with coffee, that they had to fight off Jennifer, Gwendoline, Marjorie and Brenda all at once. Each of them claimed me as her own.

What the hell was I to do?

I woke next morning with a terrible hangover and staggered down to the surgery to be met by Gladys, scowling and looking really grumpy.

'There have been four personal calls for you already this morning, Doctor Bob,' she said, handing me a list.

I didn't need to look. It was Jennifer, Gwendoline, Marjorie and Brenda.

What was I to do?

I had a week's holiday due, but where could I go to escape this lot?

Suddenly I thought of my mother. I really was being driven back to the womb. My mother had been widowed when I was three, was young and active, and led her own independent life.

We were good friends and she was always a good counsellor. She spent a great deal of her time as an active member of the Liberal Party. We wrote to each other frequently and always kept in close touch.

I rang her and explained my problem. I could hear her laughing at the other end of the phone. 'Well, Bob,' she said, 'you had better come away with your old Mum. I am off to a quiet hotel near Bournemouth for a week. Just throw a few things in your case, and come.'

I spent the remainder of the week avoiding my four admirers. Gladys was a marvel on the phone. From her answers I was out on emergencies for forty-eight hours on the trot.

Eventually I made my escape. On the Friday I sneaked out of the house and got into my car at two o'clock in the morning. I daren't travel by daylight – I was sure there would have been road blocks.

I arrived at my mother's hotel at Boscombe at eight in the morning having spent some time at an all-night cafe en route, anxiously looking out of the window to see if I had any pursuers.

I slept the whole day and made my first appearance at dinner.

My mother was young and attractive and had already made several friends in the hotel. Most were much older than I, but I had noticed a couple of girls sitting at a nearby table who were round about my age.

But did I really want ever to have anything to do with girls again?

Both these two looked very pleasant – I particularly liked the blonde one. Neither of them looked like the pack of man-eaters I had just escaped from.

We all sat round having coffee after dinner and I found the two girls were called Pam and Joan. Pam worked for an advertising magazine and Joan was a secretary in London.

Pam and I got on like a house on fire. She talked to me as if I were her Father Confessor. I had been introduced to her as

186

a 'Doctor', so perhaps that was why it was. She told me all about her broken engagement and how she had come away with a friend to try and sort herself out and forget the upsets of the last few months.

Eventually the older people went to bed. Pam looked a little bit puzzled when my mother went, and eventually Joan slipped away, leaving us sitting on the settee together.

We found we had an awful lot in common. She thought I was terribly funny and laughed at all my jokes; but there was something hesitant in her manner and if I moved a bit too close to her on the settee she would spring away as if she would have been electrocuted if I touched her.

She agreed, reluctantly, to have a game of squash with me next day. I assumed that she still was grieving over her lost fiancé. She warned me that she had never played squash before. But she was nice, easy to be with, and for once it looked as if I would have to make the move towards the opposite sex rather than the other way round.

Pam looked lovely in her squash clothes – small red shorts and a tight-fitting singlet. She really was super.

I instructed her in the rudiments of the game and then began to show off atrociously. Not to be outdone, Pam chased round after every ball I hit. I ran her almost to the point of exhaustion, but she still kept on going.

She somehow managed to return one of my smashes to the bottom left-hand corner. I leapt across the court to make yet one more impossible retrieve. As I flashed my racket back it hit something soft, and there was Pam doubled up on the floor of the squash court, not breathing, completely winded by my blow to her solar plexus.

I rushed over to her, alarmed. She really had stopped breathing. I pressed on her chest and nothing happened. Only one thing for it, I thought – mouth-to-mouth resuscitation. As my lips met hers I found her chest beginning to move. Thank God she was all right.

At this moment I looked up to see that there were at least

a dozen people in the spectators' gallery, all completely trans-
fixed by this drama taking place in front of them. It is not often
you see a prone couple in a squash court, lips and bodies
locked.

I got up and helped Pam to her feet. She was sweating
from her exhaustive running and shaken from my winding blow.
She looked terribly worried. 'Oh, Bob,' she said. 'Whatever will
your wife think?'

'My wife?' I said. 'I'm not married.'

'Well who is the lady you are with? She is Mrs Clifford, isn't
she?'

I burst out laughing.

'That's my mother, you nut.'

'Oh,' said Pam, 'I thought she looked so young and smart
– just a bit older than you – and you were man and wife.'

The rest of our holiday passed in a happy blur. We were
marvellous, humorous companions. Pam looked even better in a
two-piece bathing suit than she had done on the squash court.
This was for real – and mother liked her too.

All too soon the holiday was over and I knew this was
something I was going to follow up. Pam, unfortunately, lived
in Surrey which was many miles from our practice. I found that
my partners were tolerant about me getting away for long
weekends. When it was my turn to have a weekend off, I used
either to motor down to Leatherhead where Pam's parents
lived – when I would watch her in the amateur dramatic society
where she always seemed to play the maid – or we would
go up to my mother's and spend the weekend with her in
London.

The months soon passed.

I was to have a week's holiday over Christmas and the
New Year and Pam had promised to come to the hospital New
Year's Ball with me. She was going to meet all my hospital
friends and it was going to be the first time that we had ever
dressed up to go out together.

She emerged from my mother's bedroom looking radiant in

a red taffeta dress which highlighted her bare, slightly freckled arms.

The ball was a great success and my friends loved her. This was the girl for me.

We were dancing together as midnight struck and the New Year of 1950 was chimed in. As the old year went out I stood back, took her face in my hands, and said, 'Pam, darling, will you marry me?'

'Of course I will,' she said. 'Your mother has been dinning the duties of a G.P.'s wife into me for the last two months.'

We were soon surrounded by smiling, congratulating friends. All my old rugby mates, some of them married already, some just about to take the plunge, and some who were determined that no event such as this was ever going to interfere with their beer drinking.

Suddenly a loud voice came over the Tannoy. The music stopped and the voice of the Admiral, the lodge porter who had been at the hospital for at least thirty years, who had been a father and uncle and just about everything to all of us at some time or another, brought the proceedings to a halt.

'Ladies and Gentlemen,' he began, 'I would like two minutes' silence. Bob Clifford has just got engaged – one more rugby player has bitten the dust.'

Pam hugged me.

Life was going to be different from now on.

Postscript

There is the fable of the old man sitting outside a town, being approached by a stranger.

'What are they like in this town?' asked the stranger.

'What were they like in your last town?' replied the old man.

'They were delightful people. I was very happy there. They were kind, generous and would always help you in trouble.'

'You will find them very much like that in this town.'

The old man was approached by another stranger.

'What are the people like in this town?' asked the second stranger.

'What were they like in your last town?' replied the old man.

'It was an awful place. They were mean, unkind and nobody would ever help anybody.'

'I am afraid you will find it very much the same here,' said the old man.

If it should be your lot to ever visit Tadchester, this is how you will find us.